Acknowledgements

As with all good things, many are to be acknowledged for their support, encouragement, critique and hand holding in this endeavor:

- Thanks to TEC Canada, whose request for a workbook for my seminars compelled me to get this down on paper.

- To all my "lay editors", including Paul Brubaker, Kimberly Clark and Gail Olson, who helped me gooder my grammar and get rid of the typoz.

- To my bud, Cindi Zellner, who spent a memorable afternoon in the park playing photographer.

- To Kathy Conroy I'll forever by indebted for commenting, "You want people to understand it's as easy as their morning coffee..."

- And to Stephanie Wirkkala, without whom this would never have been a "real book".

As Easy As
Your Morning Coffee

Simple Steps to Fitness Success

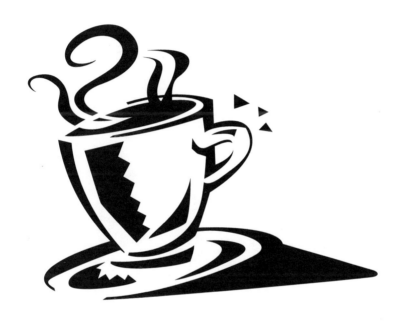

Judi Ulrey

ISBN 0-9668042-0-1

Dedication

To my Papa, who walked the extra mile to get me through college so I could pursue my dreams, whatever they may be.

Contents

Important! Read this!
(pretty please...)

Preface

The fact that you have picked up this book suggests there is a possibility you want to move in the direction of a more healthy lifestyle. If that is <u>not</u> the case, don't panic! No *commitments* required! (ugh! That "c" word!)

But bear in mind it is written with the assumption you are interested in developing some new attitudes and habits and are ready to honestly complete the suggested exercises. The goal of this project was to create a book that someone could access over and over again. When it comes to fitness programs, few people get on the band wagon and stay on. More often than not, people start a program - get distracted - start a program - get distracted - and so it goes. This book is designed to "be there for you" when you are ready to start up again. It is a back-to-the-basics, step-by-step, hold your hand guide.

Given that, my vision is that you can create a structure for your program by focusing on one chapter per week. That way you are not trying to make too many changes at one time, but instead are adding one new health habit at a time. If you prefer to add one habit per month, that's ok too. Also, do the chapters in any order you wish. It is very flexible. The process is yours to choose.

With one exception. Step Number One.

Positive Mental Attitude really is the first and most important step. A positive attitude gets you 70% down the road. And trying to focus on any of the other steps before working on your thoughts will be exceptionally challenging.

I believe each of the 12 steps is important. If I didn't, they would not be included in the book.

At the same time, there is benefit to pursuing *any one habit,* even if you never conquer them all. It is **not** an all-or-nothing program. I have identified 12 behaviors that if done regularly will dramatically improve your health and well-being. But some steps are certainly better than no steps. If you conquer even one step, good for you! You will do them when you are ready.

So why haven't I mentioned smoking?

I am very pleased to watch the smoking population rapidly diminish. In the U.S. we went from 51.9% male smokers and 33.9% female in 1965 to 27.7% of the men and 25% women in 1993.* Halleluia!

But for those of you who have not kicked the nasty habit, may I go on record:

> ## Smoking is the #1 **WORST**** thing you can do to your health.

Choosing to be smoke free is <u>critical</u> to good health. But because this is not an issue for the vast majority of the population, we will not address it in this book. But for you hangers-on, (Dad...) I encourage you to contact your physician or healthcare provider for assistance in kicking the habit. And **kudos to you!** for taking that step!

Fitness

The word "fitness" can conjure up a multitude of misleading visions. Think of "fit" people and what comes to mind?

- young
- thin
- pretty
- "perfectly happy"
- brainless baboons

A condition that not only seems unattainable but possibly compulsive, abnormal, and boring.

Fit is defined as "sound physically and mentally; healthy".

Fitness is the quality or state of being healthy.

Nothing is mentioned about <u>perfect</u> weight, <u>perfect</u> body, Super Stud! So why do we have these misconceptions?

* Source: American Lung Assn.
**Worst: Bad or ill in the extreme degree; most unsatisfactory or objectionable; most injurious; most unpleasant, unattractive, or disagreeable. (Get the message?!?)

An Apology

On behalf of my industry, <u>please accept our apology.</u>

In the first half of this century we moved without giving it much thought. We worked in the garden, did the wash by hand, carried water from the well, and danced to Benny Goodman.

During the '60's we got our exercise by marching through campus holding signs. (And sometimes running from police.)

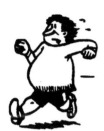 Then in the '70's a guy from Dallas came along and says, "You can't just march, you gotta RUN!" No pain - No gain!

And on the band wagon many jumped.

By the 80's we were getting our aerobic points via "aerobics".

(Look that one up in your Funk & Wagnalls...)

[Funk & Wagnalls! Are they still around?? What ever happened to ol' "Funk"? And good ol' Wagnalls, what a great guy...]

Oh, sorry. Brain stray. It happens... Back to aerobics...

"Step - ball - change... turn right... do-si-do... now **march!** 2-3-4!"

(There's that marching thing again!)

"Now **STOP!!** Take your pulse...ready?...count!........"

If you didn't feel 25 beats or more, YOU'RE NOT WORKING HARD ENOUGH!!

"Keep marching!"

Meanwhile, 80% of the population from the vantage point of their living room couch is saying, "That sure doesn't look like fun! No wonder they call it a 'work out'! Count me out!"

And back they went to see what was on the tube.

A note of interest:

Funk & Wagnalls, a publishing firm long associated with reference books and other non-fiction, was originally founded in New York City in 1875 by Isaac K. Funk; it became Funk & Wagnalls two years later after Adam Willis Wagnalls became a partner in the enterprise. Both founders were Lutheran ministers. During its early years the company published periodicals and religious books for the clergy. A major undertaking was the publication in 1894 of *A Standard Dictionary of the English Language*. The Funk & Wagnalls Standard Encyclopedia was first published in 1912.

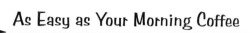

So here we are nearing the next millennium, when everything else in the world is getting *faster* (450 Mhz blah, blah), and the fitness industry is now starting to slow down.

The Surgeon General recommended in 1996 "moderate movement most days", and included gardening as one of our options. Gardening! Who'da thunk! Sure beats that marching!

So please accept our apology for leading you astray. Fitness need **not** be so hard. It truly can be *as easy as your morning coffee*.

In fact, "fitness: being in good physical condition or health" should be a <u>good</u> thing!

So please do not misread the intentions of this book. We are not promoting the Simple Steps to Becoming SuperMan/Woman.

> # We are interested in health — physical well-being.

Consider some of the following words and see if any of them speak to you:

Health - soundness of body & mind; vigor

Vitality - exuberant physical strength or mental vigor

Robust - strong & healthy; hardy; vigorous

Well-being - a state characterized by health, happiness & prosperity

Alive - full of life; lively; active; vibrant; full of verve, animation

Exercise

Choose a word, or several words, that describe the physical condition you are desiring.

Keep a Journal

I encourage you to document your thoughts <u>outside</u> this book because as I mentioned earlier, one of the real benefits of this program is you can go through it again and again. Unless you are Mr. or Ms. SuperFit, chances are you will benefit from re-reading, re-considering, re-evaluating and re-grouping from time to time. Thus, keeping a journal outside this book makes sense. (Unless, of course, you want to buy <u>several </u>copies!)

And you will change. You may want to focus on different steps at different times. The beauty of the program is it's flexibility. The steps need not be taken in any particular order, can be considered individually, and can be revisited at any time.

Are you sure you want to read this?

Before we get started, let's determine if you really <u>want</u> to. I mean, why spend the time? You could just as easily spend your personal time watching a soap, reading a good book, or taking a nap. Right? So why bother?

As mentioned previously, this book was written for people who have decided it is time to change some habits to better their health. But we all know how unmotivating it is to do something just because "it's good for you". Is that the only reason you are pursuing this? Are you doing it under duress? (prodded by a concerned spouse, parent, child, etc.?) Are there reasons YOU want to make changes in your lifestyle? Do you see benefits to making changes? Take a moment to honestly assess <u>your</u> motives (not someone elses...).

List all the things you perceive to be benefits to making healthy lifestyle choices, **AND** the real-life, got-to-consider, "it's-a-hassle" drawbacks. Typical entries for each side are provided.

+		-	
8	weight control	2	sweat - UGH!

So how did you do?

Did your **+** list outweigh your **-** list? Is it a pretty close call?   Well, just to make sure, let's rate the significance of each of the benefits and drawbacks on a scale of 1-10.

1 = very **in**significant

10 = very, very significant

For example, a benefit of developing a healthy lifestyle might be the positive role model for your family or your employees, and that is a 9-10 significance. A disadvantage of healthy choices is you sweat when you exercise, and that's stinky. But honestly, in the grand scheme of things, maybe that's not truly significant, so you rate it a 2. Go back and rate each issue.

So how do your column tallies compare? Does the benefits side outweigh the drawbacks? Dramatically? So <u>objectively</u>, healthy lifestyle choices make sense, huh?

So why are they so difficult to sustain? — Lots of reasons.

#1 Lack of Time

With all the new toys and technology, theoretically we are significantly more efficient today than ever in history. So why are we all still working so hard? Why can't we accomplish what we need to accomplish in a 20 hour work week? Why are we still complaining we need 25 hours in a day? That is a discussion in human psychology and sociology, which is outside the realm of this book, but suffice it to say, we <u>choose</u> to be very busy, so time for self care is at a minimum.

#2 Lack of Support

Despite today's focus on healthy lifestyles and well-living, society actually is **unsupportive** of personal health.

Consider Fast Food restaurants. Until the 1950's, we didn't have the option of *insta-fat via the drive thru*. But today, every major intersection supports a fast food restaurant alluring the busy public to consume on-the-run. And consider life's pace today. There was a time in our not-so-distant history that our communication with others took weeks. Today, 1-2 days with "snail mail" is totally unacceptable (not to mention the inconvenience of posting a stamp...).

#3 Lack of a Plan

One reason physical success so frequently eludes people is **lack of planning.** An effective exercise program needs a strategic plan determining the what, when and where. Eating healthfully requires one to shop for the necessary staples, and do a bit of meal planning. But we seem to plan for our kids soccer season or our business needs, and leave our health habits to chance. To ensure success, you need a Health Plan.

Ask someone if they have a Health Plan, and they will likely respond, "Sure. I am with an HMO.", or "Yes, I have health benefits through my employer", or "Of course, I would never go without a Health Plan". But the question is not "Do you have Medical Insurance?" It is –

Do you have a Health Plan?

A Health Plan is a personal program for the promotion of long term health. It is a plan for **preventing** injury and disease - to keep you vibrant and alive. Yet all too often we plan our social calendar far more attentively than our health. And when it's gone, regret abounds.

The simple steps that follow provide you a format for developing a Health Plan. But Buyer Beware: It is **NOT** a quick fix! It is a program encouraging you to make small but hopefully permanent changes in your lifestyle. It is about developing more healthy habits that will make you feel better and have more energy and probably lose fat. But it's not an instant solution to anything. It's a tool to use and reuse and reuse as you choose to take good care of yourself during this life's journey.

Are you ready?

Let's go!!

Judi Ulrey
Fitness Consulting, Inc.
Fall 1998

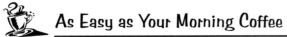

The Buddy System

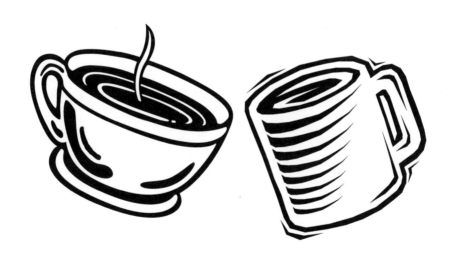

Get a Buddy

Regardless of your enthusiasm for your renewed commitment to a more healthy lifestyle, you will have days you want to punt! There will be times when you **don't** want to exercise, you want to eat potato chips rather than veggies, and you have a **bad** attitude! Welcome to the roller coaster of life.

But you can shorten those peaks and valleys with a buddy - a pal with whom you can share your process, your progress, your feelings and your frustrations. This person can help to motivate you when you are not, encourage you when you are down, and applaud your successes. **All** very important jobs!

So what's a Buddy to do?

Whatever you need him/her to do. But the important thing is expectations must be **clear**.

Some Buddy examples:

Exercise Buddy - Someone who commits to walk/exercise with you once, twice, three times per week.

Accountability Buddy - Someone with whom you share your exercise log on a weekly basis. Just knowing you are accountable to someone improves motivation. (Funny how that works...)

Phone Buddy - Someone you can call, any time, for encouragement.

Can you think of others?

List them here:

_____

_____

_____

_____

_____

Buddy Contracts

Committing an intention to writing **always** heightens the obligation. It is a bilateral agreement that clarifies the responsibilities of both parties.

Take a look at the chapter's end.

In fairness to all parties, Buddy Contracts should be as explicit as possible. Expectations must be clearly understood by both parties, so no one's feelings are hurt down the road.

"You promised you'd walk with me twice a week!"

"No I didn't. I said I would walk with you whenever I could."

"You aren't supporting me in this process!"

"I told you I would walk with you when I can make the time.
What more do you want from me?!?" ...

And so it goes.

So you see, if you choose to make a contract, **YOU MUST TAKE IT SERIOUSLY!!** It can be a wonderful, mutually beneficial arrangement for all.   But if not executed with care, can be a source of disillusionment.

Make a list of the ways in which you would like to be supported.

1. _____
   _____

2. _____
   _____

3. _____
   _____

4. _____
   _____

5. _____
   _____

6. _____
   _____

7. _____
   _____

8. _____
   _____

9. _____
   _____

10. _____
    _____

Recruitment List

Make a list of those people who would sincerely be interested in supporting you.

1. _____

   _____

2. _____

   _____

3. _____

   _____

4. _____

   _____

5. _____

   _____

6. _____

   _____

(This is a terrific exercise, because even if you do not recruit all these people to help you with your health program, look at all those who <u>love</u> you! If you think they would be *willing* to support you, they must love you!)

Create Your Team

OK, you've identified the areas in which you would like to have some support. You have your recruitment list. Now create your team! Having a broad based, multi-person support team makes your process easier and more fun. Your Exercise Buddy may not be your best Food Coach. You likely will want support both at home and at work. Out of towners can help via phone or e-mail. You might even want to hire a personal trainer or food coach. You don't want to make this overly complicated by enlisting a veritable army, but **community** support is good.

Warning: Buddies may Bail

Take care not to put all your eggs in your Buddy's basket. "To err is human...", so you just may have a buddy bail on you. Don't let this disrupt your process, nor should you allow yourself to use it as an excuse. Remember, your bestest buddy is <u>yourself</u>. True change comes from within. Appreciate and enjoy any and all support you receive from others, but if they don't come through like you expected, forgive and move on.

Team Roster

<u>Friend</u>   <u>will support me by</u>

1. _____

2. _____

3. _____

4. _____

5. _____

6. _____

7. _____

Buddy Contract

(sample)

Whereas inactivity has been determined to be a primary risk factor for heart disease, many cancers, stroke and diabetes, and

Whereas I _____Jane Doe_____ am committed to be a positive role model for my family/
(you)

organization, and

Whereas I, _____Jane Doe_____ desire to live a quality life, unrestrained by physical
(you)

limitations, I pledge to ___walk 3 times per week for a minimum of 30 minutes per session___
(area in which you want to be supported)

Furthermore

Whereas I, _____Sue Ray_____ am highly interested in the well-being of
(buddy)

_____Jane Doe_____ and am committed to support him/her in any way
(you)

possible, I pledge to:

1) accompany her on her walks a minimum of 2x/week

2) review her exercise card every week during our 10:00 a.m. break

3) refrain from bringing unhealthy foods (like Haagen Dazs ice cream...) into our home

4) be available by phone at any time to encourage and support him in his personal health process

Buddy Contract

Whereas inactivity has been determined to be a primary risk factor for heart disease, many cancers, stroke and diabetes, and

Whereas I _____ am committed to be a positive role model for my family/
(you)
organization, and

Whereas I, _____ desire to live a quality life, unrestrained by physical
(you)
limitations, I pledge to _____
(area in which you want to be supported)

Furthermore

Whereas I, _____ am highly interested in the well-being of
(buddy)
_____ and am committed to support him/her in any way
(you)
possible, I pledge to:

1) accompany her on her walks a minimum of 2x/week

2) review her exercise card every week during our 10:00 a.m. break

3) refrain from bringing unhealthy foods (like Haagen Dazs ice cream...) into our home

4) be available by phone at any time to encourage and support him in his personal health process

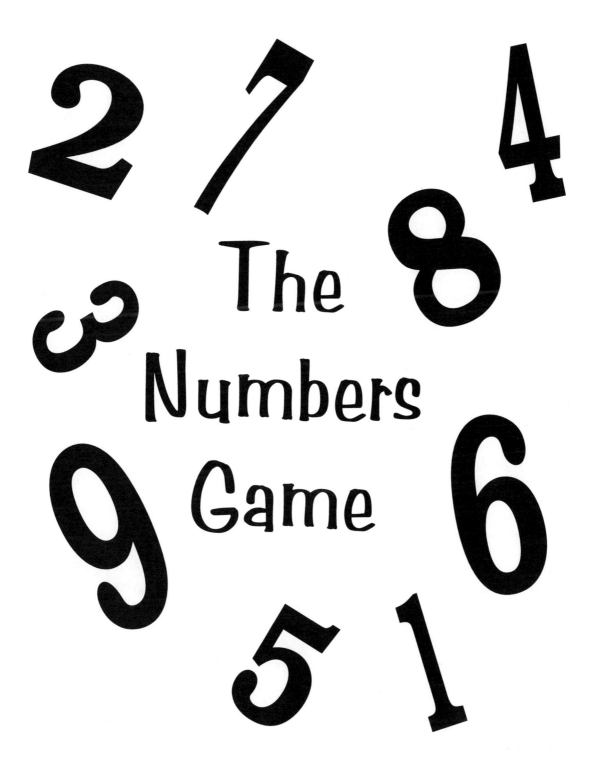

The Numbers Game

The Numbers Game

This next chapter is for all you accountant-types and numbers people. If you like a program that allows you to monitor your progress with charts and graphs and statistics, then this one's for you.

All too often when people start a fitness program, they have one singular goal in mind: to lose weight. They don't look at their reduction in blood pressure. They don't consider the benefits of muscular development. They don't acknowledge or even monitor lowering their cholesterol.

They simply want to **lose weight**.

I honestly think some people would consider cutting off an appendage just so the scale weight would go down. Or just as ridiculous, get their fat sucked off with liposuction. Not too smart.

Health and fitness is a much bigger issue than just weight. So look at the Big Picture. Consider all your physical statistics that are improving.

Get Off the Scale

This program is so much not about weight, I challenge you to throw out your bathroom scale. It is a useless tool. And it taints your perspective.

Body Fat Percentage should be your concern.

Experts recommend that women carry no more than 22-25% body fat and men 15-18%. That means no more than 22%/15% of total body weight should come from fat, with 78%/85% being lean weight - bones, muscle, organs and body fluids. Unfortunately, American women average around 36% and men are bulging at 26%. So as a population, we are over fat.

> # But the scale can't tell you if you've lost fat!

Go on a crazy starvation diet, surviving on carrots and celery (and an occasional binge...) and you likely will lose muscle weight.

A True Story About Theresa

Several years ago Fitness Consulting coordinated a fat loss contest at a small company. About 40 employees had their body fat tested. We then divided them into two teams, so the average body fat on each team and the mix of men to women was approximately the same. Over a 10-week period, the <u>team</u> that lost the most body fat won.

Enter Theresa.

Theresa arrived for her second body fat test. Enthusiastically, I asked, "So Theresa, how did you do?"

Very sheepishly she answered, "Well...ok."

Not very convincing.

She proceeded to tell me she had lost 10 pounds, (*"Great!!"*) but that she was confounded, as her clothes weren't fitting any differently. (*"Uh oh...Not so great..."*) When someone loses 10 pounds of fat, their clothes will be falling off.

So we put Theresa in the hydrostatic weighing tank, and got the bad news. She was fatter than when she started. She had lost 8 pounds of muscle, and only 2 pounds of fat!

<u>Note</u>: The scale had been telling her she was making great progress. She had lost 10 pounds! When in fact, her body fat percentage was increasing by the day.

So very gently I inquired, "So Theresa, tell me about your exercise program."

"I've been riding my bicycle for 30 minutes every day."

Good.

"And...what have you been eating?!?"

And off she rambled, identifying "a bite of this" and "a bite of that", "a half cup of cereal" and "a handful of ..."

I calculated she had been consuming a mere 600-700 calories/day.

She had been starving herself.

So her body had been storing fat in self defense, and had lost muscle.

The dieters dilemma.

So after the tears, (hers, not mine) I explained to Theresa that her body <u>needs food</u> to survive, and any time she dramatically reduces her calories (less than 1200 for women, 1500 for men) her body thinks it is being starved, stores fat in self defense, and goes to the protein in her muscle mass for fuel.

I recommended she <u>double</u> her caloric intake, (she couldn't believe it - she was supposed to be dieting!) and continue to ride her bike every day.

8 weeks pass.

Theresa comes back to check her body fat. And this time she's <u>really</u> confused.

When I asked about her progress she reported, "I haven't lost an ounce!! But look at these baggy jeans!"

She jumped in the tank and my hypothesis proved true.

This time with the combination of exercise and the correct number of quality calories, Theresa gained 6 pounds of muscle, (6 of the 8 she had lost the first time around...) and lost 6 pounds of fat!! The scale told her she was slacking - "hadn't lost an ounce" - when in fact she had lost 2% body fat!

So how do I measure my body fat?

There are lots of new-fangled machines on the market, many of which are only marginally accurate.

Hydrostatic, or under water weighing, is still considered the most accurate means of measuring body fat. Because fat floats and bones and muscles sink in water, by expelling as much air from your lungs as you can and "dunking" under water, you can accurately test your body fat. You will likely need to contact a local community college or university to find a tank.

Skin calipers are also very popular, and much more readily accessible. With calipers a consultant will "pinch an inch" of fat at 3-6 different sites on your body and from there calculate body fat. Many health clubs offer skin caliper testing.

So the message is, punt your scale!! Begin concentrating on your muscle/fat weight ratio.

Other important numbers

Because you will be making improvements in a variety of areas, you will want to keep track of them all. It gives you more opportunities to pat yourself on the back!

A Tougher Ticker

So you also want to improve your cardiovascular fitness, eh? How will you know if you are?

Check out these numbers:

Resting Heart Rate

Remember, the stronger your heart is, the more blood it distributes with every beat, so the less often it needs to beat. Slower is better.

What is your resting heart rate first thing in the morning? (assuming you didn't wake up to a house fire or earthquake...)

Don't know?

Let's check it now.

Touch both your index and middle fingers either on your wrist, along your thumb line, or on your carotid artery on your neck. (Don't press too hard on the carotid - you could pass out.)

Feel it?

Now start counting.

Count for 15 seconds, then multiply that number by 4.

That's your resting heart rate.

Start keeping track of that number regularly in the morning.

The more consistent your exercise, the lower your pulse.

Recovery Rate

Here's another test of the strength of your heart.

Get out and do your normal aerobic exercise.

Walk. Run. Ride a bicycle.

After 15-30 minutes, start your cool down, slowing your pace, but <u>do not stop!</u> (Stopping abruptly could cause you to get dizzy and faint.)

Three minutes into your cool down, check your pulse.

This is your **Recovery Rate**.

The stronger your heart is, the more quickly it will recover!

So keep track of your Recovery Rate, watching your heart gradually slow down more and more quickly after exercise. That is another sign your heart is getting stronger! Yet another reason to pat yourself on the back!

VO2

VO2 is the volume of oxygen your heart can distribute through your system during exercise. The stronger it is, the more oxygen it can distribute.

To determine VO2, you must do an exercise test on a calibrated treadmill or bicycle. How does your heart respond to varying workloads on the bicycle? If an easy workload really skyrockets your heart rate, that suggests your heart is not very efficient. Conversely, if your heart is good and strong, it will require an extremely difficult workload to elevate it. From assessing these heart rates relative to workloads, we can determine VO2. You will probably need to find either a health club that offers the test, or a university fitness testing lab. It is called a graded exercise test.

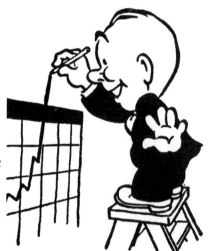

Regardless, you can measure Resting Heart Rate and Recovery Rate on your own.

Remember, these numbers are only a fingertip away.

Strength and Flexibility

Though strength and flexibility testing are a bit primitive, monitoring is better than not monitoring.

If you currently never stretch and can barely reach your toes, and you start a stretching program and within 8 weeks can stretch two inches beyond your toes, wouldn't you call that significant? But you would never know you had progressed unless you had tested yourself.

Oftentimes consultants use a sit-and-reach box to test flexibility. It is literally a yardstick-on-a-box. You can make your own by gluing a yardstick on a box. Place your feet on the sides of the box and slowly bend forward. How far along the yardstick can you reach? Now watch your progress.

And the same goes for strength testing.

If today you can barely do one full push up, but over a period of time you improve to 10 push-ups, wouldn't you call that progress? And if you can only "stomach" 10 crunches* when you start your program, and slowly progress to 100 crunches/day, your abs are abs • olutely getting stronger! So keep track. It is motivational! Again, more reasons for giving yourself a pat on the back.

* Never do the old fashioned full sit-up. Instead, look up to the ceiling with your hands supporting your head and <u>using your abdominal muscles</u> raise your shoulders 4-6" off the ground.

Cholesterol

We will be discussing the significance of cholesterol later, but it should be mentioned here as one of the statistics you will want to monitor. If you don't check it, how will you know if it is getting better??

Fitness Record

Following is a Fitness Record on which you can make entries of blood pressure, resting heart rate, recovery rate, push-ups, sit-ups and sit-and-reach. (The weight entry is optional.)

Keeping this log current will give you a format for consistently monitoring your physical progress in all the key areas.

Remember: Keeping track keeps you accountable!

FITNESS RECORD FOR _____

	Goal Weight	Actual Weight	Goal BC	Actual BC	Goal B.P.	Actual B.P.	Goal RHR	Actual RHR	Goal RR	Actual RR	Goal VO2	Actual VO2	Goal Chol.	Actual Chol.	Goal Risk Ratio	Actual Risk Ratio	Goal Push Ups	Actual Push Ups	Goal Sit Ups	Actual Sit Ups	Goal Scr•Reach	Actual Scr•Reach
January																						
February																						
March																						
April																						
May																						
June																						
July																						
August																						
September																						
October																						
November																						
December																						

Fitness Record Key: Weight Optional, B.C. = Body Composition, B.P. = Blood Pressure,
RHR = Resting Heart Rate, RR = Recovery Rate, VO2 = Aerobic Capacity, Chol. = Cholesterol

Exercise

Make an appointment for your first fitness evaluation. Your best bet for finding a testing lab is either a health club, or a university or community college with a degree program in Exercise Science, Exercise Physiology, or Kinesiology. Remember, you are looking for a body fat test, graded exercise test, and strength and flexibility assessment. You may be able to have the blood lipid panel done there also, or you may need to access your healthcare provider for that piece. Then commit to a semi-annual evaluation, <u>forever</u>. The January/July schedule is always a good one. (Keeps you honest during the Holidays...) This consistent "look" helps you progress toward your goals, and from straying too far once you have achieved them.

Step #1

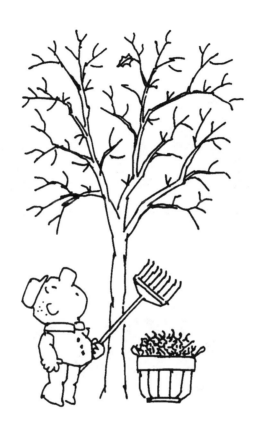

Be Positive!

Move

your

Mind.

It's All in Your Head

Entire books have been written on the impact of attitude on outcome.

Our intention here is not to rival Robert Schuller or Norman Vincent Peale. But, as I mentioned in the preface, Attitude Counts! In any of life's endeavors, whether or not you believe you will be successful, you will be right. To be successful you must _believe_ in yourself. Yet how many times have you started an exercise or food program and heard yourself say:

"I never finish these type of programs."

"I'll try it, but I've never been successful."

"Nothing ever works for me."

"I've always been heavy. I think I'm just destined to be fat."

And even after you have made some progress...

"I think I'll keep my 'fat clothes', just in case I gain back the weight."

Then guess what...

Sound familiar?

What are some of your favorite negative phrases?

_____

_____

_____

_____

_____

You can change your tapes

But what if you really <u>don't</u> believe you will be successful? You've tried everything and you just can't seem to get the results you want.

First, analyze the results you want.

Are they realistic?

A True Story About Nancy

One morning about 5:00 my phone rang. It was Nancy. Crying. Crying hysterically.

I was frantic. Was something wrong with one of her children? Was she all right?

"Nancy! Talk to me! What's wrong?! Tell me what's wrong!"

Sob... Sniff...   Snort...

"I'm so <u>slow</u>!"

Pause, while Judi regroups...

"What?!"

"I'm so <u>slow</u>!"

Then she proceeded to tell me she had been preparing for a 2-mile "predicted run competition", where everyone runs two miles, and the person completing the run in the time <u>closest to what s/he had predicted</u> wins the race. She had just run the course, had projected she would run it in 20 minutes, and it had taken her 24+.

About this she's hysterical?! And for this she has awakened me at 5:00am!?!

"So Nancy," I say, trying to exude patience, "What made you <u>think</u> you would run a 10-minute mile?"

Pause...

"I don't know..." sniff...sniff...

She had picked the number "10-minute mile" **from the air**, attached it to her heart and soul, and beat herself to a <u>pulp</u> for not attaining that unrealistic goal.

Sound familiar? Ever set yourself up for failure by having totally unrealistic expectations? Then <u>pummel</u> yourself for not reaching it?

So, back to you not believing in your own success. Have you had realistic expectations??

Next, when you are <u>sure</u> you have set some truly attainable goals, <u>*decide to believe.*</u>

"But I just don't know if I can do it?!"

Tell yourself you can.

"Lie to myself?"

No, <u>convince</u> yourself.

Aspire Higher

All too often we limit ourselves by our negative thinking.

Do you think Michael Jordan questions his ability to dunk a basketball?

Does Harrison Ford question whether or not he will be able to act a particular role?

Or do you think Michelangelo wondered, "But what if people don't like my work?!"

No!

Success requires you to proceed with confidence.

And if you lack that confidence, talk yourself into it!

Your self talk either works for you, or against you, so get it on your side!!

Affirmations are defined as "a confirmation; an assertion of the truth or existence of something" And research reveals that people who think positively - who affirm themselves and their own actions - are not only happier, but are more likely to reach their goals.

So when those doubts arise (and they will), combat them with positive affirmations.

33

We also can be negative by approaching a new program
only in terms of what we must give up:

"I need to lose weight"

"I have to quit eating my favorite foods."

"I have to give up my lunch hour to exercise."

In this program we are going to focus on what we are **getting**.

Remember all those **benefits** you identified?

Turn each benefit into an affirmation, and post them clearly in a visible place.

"I am learning new recipes that give me energy AND taste great."

"I am increasing my energy so I feel better throughout the day."

"During my exercise I get time to be alone, rejuvenate and de-stress."

Write you own affirmations.

1. _____
_____

2. _____
_____

3. _____
_____

4. _____
_____

5. _____
_____

6. _____
_____

7. _____
_____

8. _____
_____

9. _____
_____

10. _____
_____

Dreaming It True

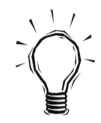

All things start as a thought.

"What if we created a vehicle that was self propelled, moving people from place to place faster than horses," dreamed Henry Ford.

"What if we created a flying machine that could travel faster than automobiles, and could fly over the great oceans?" fantasized the Wright Brothers.

"What if we could transfer written documentation via telephone lines," envisioned the first maker of the FAX.

"What if we created a telephone system using radio waves," speculated the cellular phone developers.

If you can <u>dream</u> it, you can do it, be it, or have it.

So let's take some time, dreaming, describing and documenting the physical condition to which you aspire.

Describe the activities in which you want to participate without physical limitations.

_____

_____

_____

_____

_____

_____

_____

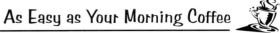

Describe the physical condition and lifestyle to which you aspire. Now be realistic!
Consider the "numbers" described in the intro.

_____

_____

_____

_____

_____

_____

_____

List as many adjectives as possible that describe your desired physical condition and
lifestyle.

_____

_____

_____

_____

_____

_____

Morning Mantra

What are you telling yourself in the morning?

"Today's going to be tough."

"I dread going to work."

"Ugh, I have to go to such & such meeting..."

Guess what? You have set yourself up for a bad day.

Sometimes it is difficult to genuinely be enthused about the day ahead... same old routine... work... have to's...

Regardless, making your morning thoughts positive, even if you must <u>read a script</u> because joy is not gushing from your soul, **read it**. Say it. Think positive. Look on the bright side. It will make you feel better, which will make you feel better.

Following are some **affirmations** to get you started on the right track in the morning.

"Today I will relax as I purposefully move from task to task."

"I will enjoy and appreciate the people with whom I come in contact today."

"I will take deep breaths regularly throughout this day."

"Today is a new adventure!"

"Traffic doesn't bother me. It gives me time to think."
(Whew! That's a tough one to swallow!)

"Today I will be conscious and accepting of the world around me."

Step #2

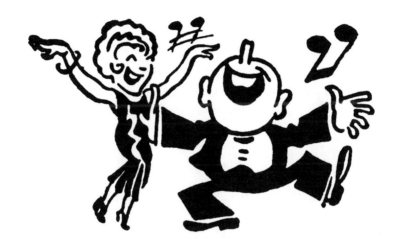

Keep Movin'

One wise marketeer once said,

Just do it.

And profound that was.

The bad news is in the summer of 1996, the Surgeon General officially announced **inactivity** to be a risk factor for heart disease, many cancers, stroke, and diabetes. Our sedentary lifestyle is killing us.

The good news, however, is we simply have to _move_ to lower our risk. We don't have to stress and strain and huff and puff. So taking time to walk each day, in addition to releasing some stress, lowers your risk of fatal disease. And the Surgeon's challenge is moderate movement **most** days. (Mathematicians concluded that in a 7 day week, that's at least 4...)

Let's look at some numbers.

Theoretically, your **maximum heart rate**, above which you should not go, is:

$$\boxed{220 \text{ - Age}}$$

So if you are 40 years old, your maximum heart rate is:

$$220 \text{ - } 40 = 180 \text{ b.p.m.}$$

B.P.M. is beats per minute. So at 40, you should not elevate your heart rate to a level above 180 beats per minute. And trust me, you don't want to! That is very strenuous!

O.K. So now we know your maximum heart rate. So?!?

Well, elevating your heart rate to varying percentages of that maximum accomplish different goals.

Check out Table 1.

Heart Rate Levels
for
40 Year Person

50-60% (of maximum)	90-108 b.p.m.	Health
60-70%	108-126	Fat Burning
70-85%	126-153	Cardiovascular
85+%	153+	Training

Table 1

If you move to the point where your heart rate is 50-60% of your maximum, you have met the requirements for lowering your risk of disease! Bravo! You see, it truly is as easy as your morning coffee! A brisk walk is all you need to do.

Now if you move a little faster, getting your heart rate to 60-70% of maximum, you will burn fat a bit more efficiently. So if you are trying to both improve your general health AND get rid of a little body fat, you will want to "step it up" to 60-70%.

Now for all of you fitness buffs who aspire to good or excellent cardiovascular fitness, creating an efficient, strong cardiovascular system, you have got to pump even harder. For cardiovascular training, elevate your HR (heart rate) to 70-85% max. Now you are starting to huff and puff. This feels like a 7 or 8 on a scale of 1-10. (See Perceived Exertion Chart) If you haven't been exercising regularly, DON'T START HERE!! This is for those who have been moving awhile.

And finally, serious athletes will train at 85%+. Their aspirations go well beyond basic health maintenance and into performance. Most people need not exercise at such a high intensity.

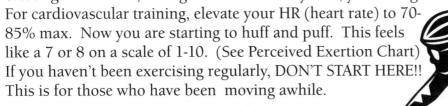

Exercise Duration and Frequency,

otherwise known as

"How long do I gotta do this?"

Before going into prescribed guidelines for exercise duration, take note:

ANYTHING IS BETTER THAN NOTHING.

If the guidelines say walk for 30 minutes, and you can only go 15, **GO 15!**

ANY PHYSICAL MOVEMENT IS BETTER THAN NONE!

And studies are revealing comparable benefit to two 15-minute walks
as to one 1/2 hour session.

Any time you get your body out moving it is very happy!

Perceived Exertion

Several studies have been done on the amazing correlation between people's subjective rating of exercise intensity and true intensity as a percentage of theoretical maximum heart rate. Time and time again researchers have put participants on exercise bicycles or treadmills, brought them to a predetermined intensity level, say 70%, asked the participant to rate it's difficulty on a 1-10 scale, and invariably they say "7". Elevate them to 80-85% of max, and they rate it an 8. So the message is, if you are not interested in monitoring your own heart rate during exercise, rely on your perceived exertion. For health purposes, move at a level 5-6, for fat burning 6-7, and cardiovascular improvement, 7-8.

Exercise Duration and Frequency

Now having said that, following are some guidelines:

50-60% for Health	20-30 minutes most days
60-70% for Fat Burning	30 minutes most days
70-80% for Cardio	12-30 minutes alternate days
80-90% for Training	per training schedule

Table 1

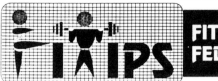

FITIPS FEBRUARY 1998

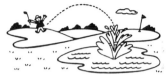

The Inside Story

You're interested in increasing the strength and effeciency of your heart, huh? So you have started exercising regularly. Walking. Cycling. Swimming. Your heart's a pumpin'.

How fast? Do you know?

Remember in September of last year we discussed the physical impact of various intensities of aerobic exercise? (See chart below) Lower intensity is great for general health improvement and fat burning. Higher intensity is what you need to strengthen the heart to higher levels. So your exercise heart rate is significant!

But how do you measure?

Well, if you can count past 10 (get a partner if you need extra fingers and toes...) you can test it manually. Feel your pulse for 10 seconds and multiply by 6. (Remember, the minute you stop exercising your pulse starts to slow down.)

But if you have trouble walking and counting (not to mention chewing gum...) there's an easier way. Get a pulse monitor.

Pulse monitors come in a variety of shapes and sizes but the ones with a chest strap and digital watch are the most accurate. Put on the chest strap and watch your watch. It's that easy.

But why do you care about your pulse rate?

Actually, it provides you with some very valuable information. First, is your workout working? Remember the goal is to strengthen your heart muscle. The stronger it is the less often it has to beat. So as you venture out week after week doing the same exercise regimen, is your exercise heart rate declining? That's because your heart's getting stronger! That's good news! (Now the bad news is if you want to maintain that exercise HR you will have to work harder.)

It also is a terrific motivation tool. Maybe you have a tendency to "stroll" through your walks. If you commit to staying in a fat burning (60-70%) vs. general health (50-60%) range, you will need to push yourself a little harder.

Or if you are on an exercise bike - again - and it's a little boring - still - do one minute sprints. What does that do to your HR? And for all of you go-getters who are pushing yourself to the limit every day, what is your HR? If you are entering the cardio training zone daily, you are likely over training.

A pulse monitor is also great for monitoring those activities that may or may not be considered aerobic exercise. Like golf. Wear a pulse monitor during your game and see the rate fluctuations. You will probably note, however, that your HR does not sustain an elevated level. (Interesting note: What happens to your HR when you hit one into the woods...?) For all you tennis players, note the difference in your HR between a singles and a doubles match. And you basketball and racquetball players may be astounded at how high your pulse rises.

The two most popular pulse monitor makers are Polar and Cardio Sport. A basic monitor that does just that will cost $80-100. If you are interested in additional features like a stop watch, lap timing, etc., they can run as high as $200. And for you statistics nerds, you can even get a contraption that allows you to interface your pulse monitor with your computer so you can print charts and graphs. Whoa!!

Happy Monitoring!

Exercise Heart Rates
[220 - age = maximum heart rate]

50-60% max = General Health Improvement
60-70% = best Fat Burning range
70-80% = Cardiovascular Improvement
80-90% = Athletic Training

FITNESS CONSULTING INC.
Since 1985
Helping you make Healthy Habits a Lifestyle
(714) 261-2639

Exercise

OK. It's your turn.

Time to figure out your own exercise prescription.

Remember:

It must be <u>realistic.</u>

It must be <u>strategic.</u>
(appropriate given your goals)

It must be <u>fun</u>!!

What days will you exercise? _____

What time of day will you exercise? _____

At what intensity will your aerobic movement be? (heart rate) _____

How long will each session be? _____

What will you do at each session? _____

_____

_____

_____

But I just don't have time to exercise!...

If you have not been in the habit of exercising , a big hurdle in your head is very possibly,

"But I just don't have time to exercise!!!"

And understandably so.

We are busier than ever as we attempt to keep pace with new technology and sociology and heightened financial obligations.

But regardless, **your physical health is your primary concern!!**

Without it, you cannot be effective in **any** other endeavor.

So we must <u>find</u> the time.

But rather than considering it another obligation, refer back to the discussion on attitude. If you consider exercise a "have to" - a drudgery - you are handicapping yourself. You are creating more turmoil in your life.

Conversely, consider your exercise time <u>your</u> time -

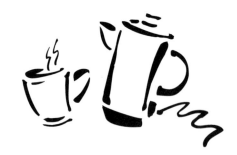

your play time -

your time to relax - and look forward to it -

just like your morning coffee.

So start with the attitude of "I am committed to <u>balance</u> in my life." I know I am a better employee, mom, student, _____, when I take time to exercise.   I look forward to my 12:30-1:30 break when I will walk with my walkman, energize my body, and prepare myself for a productive afternoon!

Following are some creative ways of incorporating exercise into your day...

Mornin' Movin'

Morning can be a time of quiet reflection and anticipation.

A new day ahead. List of things to do. Obligations to fulfill.

And what better way to prepare for maximum enjoyment and productivity than to start with some time for yourself.

Try some of the following:

10-minute morning stretch

20-minute power walk

- listen to motivating music

- visualize a productive day full of pleasant personal interactions (especially if you're going to the dentist or to see your accountant!!)

- Plan your schedule. Identify priorities; consider scheduled events; assume interruptions; schedule some down time

Take a Break!

(instrumental)

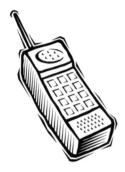

It has been a busy morning.

Phone calls. Distractions. Interruptions.

Time to re-center.

Grab your walkman.
Don your tennies.
Off you go.

For 10-minutes feel the energy of the instrumental music.

Feel the beat.

Listen to the individual sounds of the different musical instruments. Can you identify them?

If the instruments had faces/personalities, what would they be??

What adjective would you use to describe each instrument?

What feelings are aroused by this music? What memories are incited?

If you were writing a fictional story, what is happening in the story while this music is playing in the background?

Take a Break / Sing-Along

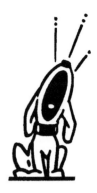

Singing is liberating.

Break out in song, and you cannot help but feel better!

Combine melody and movement and you have a <u>sure win</u>!

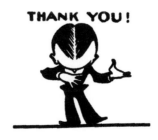

Grab your walkman with your favorite tape
of which you know the lyrics.

Off you go!

Swing those arms!

Belt out those tunes!

You will feel exhilarated, invigorated, and <u>motivated</u>!

THANK YOU!

Day's End
De-Stressor

Whew! It's been a long one!
Phones ringing.
Pagers buzzing.
Kids crying.
Bosses barking.
Employees whining.

Take a deep breath.

Take another.

One more.

Now roll those shoulders.

Change direction.

Tilt your head left.

Right.

Breathe.

Now before you jump into yet another project, take 15-30 minutes for you!

Out you go!! Around the block. Just **move.** And while you are out:

* Notice* the trees. What color are they? Describe the variations in color.

* Notice the buildings. Are the lines boxey? rounded? How are the windows of one different from its neighbor?

* What have people done to "decorate"? Do you like it? Why or why not?

* Note the people you pass. Who are they? What do they do? Speculate about their personality and lifestyle. What is their "story"?

* What do people's clothing reveal about them? Could you see yourself in the clothing styles you notice? Why? Why not?

* *Notice: to give consideration or pay attention to; heed; quiet your chatter and look around you.*

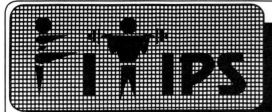

FiTips
September
1993

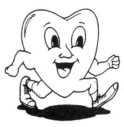

A WALK A DAY

KEEPS THE

DOCTOR AWAY!

THE WONDERS OF WALKING

Walking.   Not a new concept. Been doing it for years. So what's all the excitement about it now?? Walking is a ***fabulous*** exercise, for multiple reasons:

✓ Walking is a great way to strengthen your heart. New studies would suggest that walking 4-5 times per week will dramatically reduce your risk of cardiovascular disease.

✓ Regular walking will lower your blood pressure. Hypertension is one of the primary risk factors for heart disease, and can be moderated with exercise.

✓ Walking is a tremendous stress management tool. When you've had enough and you are ready to blow, go for a brisk walk and you're sure to feel better. This is especially true if you listen to your favorite music along the way.

✓ Walking is a terrific fat burning exercise. If you are ***serious*** about losing those extra pounds, take 30 minutes each day to **WALK!**

✓ Listen ladies: Walking is a weight bearing exercise, and therefore will reduce your risk of osteoporosis.

✓ Walking is great for socializing! Next time you want to catch up with a friend, go for a long walk instead of meeting in a restaurant or bar.

✓ You can also tone your upper body while walking. Next time you put on those walkin' shoes, grab some light dumbbells, (or baked bean cans, or detergent bottles filled with sand or water, or the two kids...) and swing those arms as you walk. This is a great upper body workout (as you will note the next day when you can't lift your arms...).

Some things to remember before you hit the pavement:

SHOES ARE IMPORTANT
Since shoes are your only equipment, it pays to invest in the right kind. Walking shoes should have a snug, well-cushioned, slightly raised heel and firm arch support. Make sure that you have adequate toe room, as your toes naturally spread as you walk. The sole should be slightly stiff and slip-resistant, but the upper more flexible, as you have more bend in your foot when walking than running.

WEAR LIGHT, COMFORTABLE CLOTHING, AND DRINK PLENTY OF WATER
In order to walk vigorously, your clothing must be loose enough to allow you to move, and light enough to allow you to breathe. Your core body temperature will naturally rise, so dress accordingly. Also, be sure to drink plenty of water before and after you exercise.

EAT BEFORE YOU EXERCISE
Your body uses carbohydrates to act as a catalyst for burning fat. You will feel much better, and burn more fat, if you have eaten something within 3 hours of your walk. (A piece of fruit or bread is fine)

WARM UP
Warm up slowly for about five minutes before your workout and gradually slow your pace before coming to a complete stop. Stretching your calf, hamstring, and quadricep muscles after your warm-up and before your walk will assist in preventing injuries. (See Bob Anderson's book, "Stretching")

So step on out!! And experience the fun of walking!

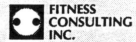

Step #3

Strength Training

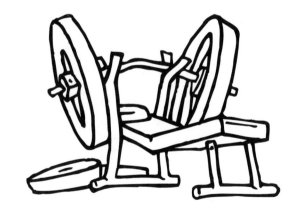

To an extent, body builders have given strength training a bad rap. When we think of lifting weights, we get a vision of a big burly guy standing in front of a mirror flexing his biceps. That is strength training taken to the extreme.

Resistance training is nothing more than exercising your muscles in order to keep them around. "Use 'em or lose 'em" is a truism. They resemble a lot of other things in life: either we pay attention to them and they serve us well, or we ignore them and they disappear.

"But", you say, "I don't really care for big, burly muscles."

That's not the point. No one's suggesting you should try to look like Arnold. But there are significant benefits to maintaining your muscle mass:

1. Structural Safety - The stronger your muscles, the less likely you are to get injured.

2. Weight Control - Muscle burns fat. The more muscle you have, the better fat burner you are.

3. Decreased Back Pain - A significant percentage of adults suffer from back pain. Back pain, strain, and injury is often a result of over exertion of weak and inflexible muscles.

4. Decreased Arthritic Pain - Strength training programs have resulted in reduction of pain for those suffering from osteoarthritis and rheumatoid arthritis.

5. Reduction in Resting Blood Pressure - Hypertension, or elevated blood pressure, is considered a primary risk factor for heart disease. Regular strength training programs have proven to reduce blood pressure.

6. Increased Bone Density - Most significantly for women who have a greater propensity for osteoporosis, strength training increases bone density.

7. Reduction in Gastrointestinal Transit Time - Strength training also reduces your risk of colon cancer, as it expedites gastrointestinal transit time.

Get the Picture?

Take a moment to consider your body.

Is it strong?

Webster defines strong as "physically vigorous or robust". It continues to expand as:

- mentally powerful or vigorous: *his mind is still strong*

- especially able, competent, or powerful in a specific field or respect: *She's very strong in mathematics.*

- of great moral power, courage, or firmness

- powerful in influence, authority, resources or means of prevailing: *a strong nation*

- compelling; of great force, effectiveness, potency or cogency: *strong arguments*

- able to resist strain, force, wear, attack, etc.: *strong walls; strong defense*

- firm or uncompromising; unfaltering

- fervent, zealous, thoroughgoing: *He's a strong Democrat.*

- strenuous or energetic; vigorous: *strong efforts*

- moving or acting with force or vigor: *strong winds*

- distinct or marked; vivid, as impressions, resemblance or contrast, etc.: *He bears a strong resemblance to his grandfather.*

- intense, as light or color.

- having a large proportion of the effective or essential properties or ingredients; concentrated: *strong tea*

and so it continues...

Do you think these qualities could be interrelated?

If one is strong physically, do you think s/he is apt to be "mentally powerful or vigorous"?

Can physical strength impact ones ability to be "powerful in influence, authority, resources or means of prevailing"?

Do you think physically strong individuals are more "strenuous or energetic, vigorous" and "able to resist strain"?

Consider your own muscular structure:

Start with your shoulders.

Then consider your chest, back, and arms.

Are they strong?

When you meet someone new and you shake their hand, is it strong? Confident? Does it suggest you are "especially able, competent, or powerful"?

Are you getting stronger each day, or weaker?

When you are 90 years old, what will you look like?

Will you stand erect - shoulders back - robust in stature?

Take a few moments visualizing yourself as strong.

This doesn't suggest looking like a body builder!

It simply means strong - robust - able to resist strain.

Exercise

Take some time to journal how having strength could impact your life, your self esteem, and/or your relationships.

_____

_____

_____

_____

_____

_____

_____

_____

_____

_____

_____

_____

_____

_____

" I got, got, got, got no time..."

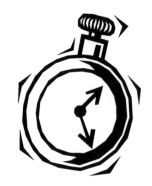

So you're busy, huh? Got no time to flex those muscles? Remember,

Maximize your Moments.

Take advantage of those few extra minutes throughout the day when you can take a break and take care of you. And if you don't have any, create them! Following are a few exercises you can do in minutes in your home or office!

Push Ups off the Desk - Just before taking off for lunch, "Do 20". Push-ups, that is.

Book Bent Over Row - Use a book for the back exercise described in <u>FiTips.</u>

Shoulder Press - Holding a book in each hand, (preferably two copies of the same book to assure equal weight) slowly press over your head. Lower to the point where your forearm is parallel to the floor. Repeat.

Triceps (back of the arm) - Securely hold a book over your head with both hands, and slowly lower behind your head, keeping your elbows close to your ears. Raise and repeat.

Lunges - Motivate your fellow employees! "Lunge" down the hallway! (Remember: Never let your knee move beyond your ankle. Lunge so your quad (thigh) and your calf make a 90 degree angle.)

Sit on the Wall - Got an extra minute? Sit on the wall! Your quadriceps will be glad you did. As mentioned in your FiTips, the Wall Sit is a great way to increase your leg strength. And you certainly have plenty of walls from which to choose! Challenge your fellow employees to a "Longest Wall Sitter" Contest!

OK, OK, you're convinced.

"But don't I have to join a gym to do strength training? I hate gyms!"

Nope. Pick up a few sets of light dumbbells and you are on your way. For under $500 you will have all the equipment you need, including a bench. The thing to remember is you want to exercise all your major muscle groups, ideally from largest muscles to smallest. Remember to take a few minutes to warm up before starting by taking a quick, brisk walk, doing jumping jacks, or simply marching in place. This gets your blood flowing and oxygen and fuel to your muscles.

NOTE: It is very difficult to demonstrate proper form via the written word. We highly recommend you work with a Fitness Professional for your first few workouts in order to learn and understand proper strength training form. Also, for those of you with "old war wounds", a Fitness Professional will work with you in developing a program taking the injury into consideration. You do <u>not</u> want to aggravate it.

So let's get started!...

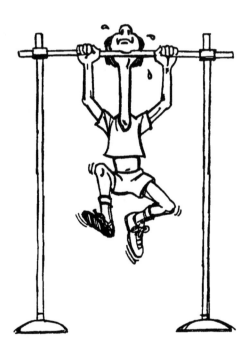

Note: For a more comprehensive reading on strength training, contact Human Kinetics at (800) 747-4457, or www.humankinetics.com. Books endorsed by ACE (American Council on Exercise) or ACSM (American College of Sports Medicine) are highly credible resources.

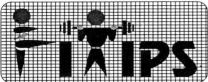 **FITIPS July 1995**

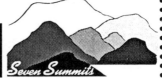
A Journey for the venturesome of spirit.

"Use 'em or Lose 'em"

So you are walking 4-5 times per week and feeling good about that, and now you are interested in toning up. But you just don't have the time (or the inclination) to get to a gym. Nor do you want to spend mega bucks on a home gym. Is there another alternative?

Absolutely! There are excellent exercises you can do at home or a work using your own body weight, and with a little imagination, you can create your own weights.

Remember that strength training is stressing your muscles beyond what they are typically accustomed. It's the "use 'em or lose 'em" principle. Either you regularly exercise them, or they slowly deteriorate, or atrophy. Unfortunately, too often the only stress our muscles get is the neck and shoulder tightness we experience from sitting at a desk all day!

So let's look at some exercises that can be easily integrated into your busy day.

Thighs

Lunges are a great exercise for the quadriceps, or front of leg. Hold each lunge for 20-30 seconds. **Remember:** Make sure your knee _never_ extends past your foot!

The wall sit is also an excellent way to increase your leg strength. With your back against the wall, as if you had a chair, support yourself solely with your legs. Time yourself, and gradually increase your time. (ouch!)

Chest

The good old fashioned push-up is a great chest exercise. If you can't do a full push-up, try it off a wall. Stand 2-3 feet away, palm on the wall. Release in and push off. Twenty push-ups takes less than a minute.

Back

Bend at the waist, soft knees, one foot in front of the other, supporting yourself with the back of a chair. Completely extend arm opposite front foot, feeling the pull of a weight (maybe a book, if you're in the office...) on your back (lats). Pull weight straight up to the side of chest, then lower. Repeat.

Shoulders

Allow weights to hang down at your thighs. Slowly raise them just short of your chin, keeping elbows out. Lower and repeat.

Then hold weights straight down at sides, palms in. With arms straight, slowly raise to shoulder height. Lower and repeat.

NOTE: Sitting in a chair while doing this exercise allows you to support your back.

Dumbbells can be purchased at any sporting goods store for about $1/pound. If you are just starting, though, use two cans of beans from your pantry. Detergent or water bottles filled with water or sand also make excellent weights. And if you are trying to integrate these exercises into your work day, bring a set to the office. You can easily complete 2-3 exercises during one of your breaks!

Triceps

Hold a weight above your head. _Carefully_ lower it behind your head, keeping your elbows close to your ears, then slowly raise again. Repeat.

Biceps

Now sit on the chair, holding a weight with palm up. Bending slightly forward and supporting your elbow on your knee, curl weight up to shoulder height. Lower and repeat.

Strength Training Tips

1. Start out slowly! You can perform any of these exercises initially with no weight at all!
2. Warm up before you start. A 3-5 minute brisk walk would be ideal, but at minimum, stretch before beginning.
3. Though the exercises look pretty straight forward, it is smart to get a professional to start you on your first program. Just let him or her know you want a program you can do at home.
4. Be cognisant of previous injuries. _Never_ work through the pain.
5. Don't forget to breath! Your muscles need the oxygen to do the work.

And have fun! Strength training is a key ingredient to better health!

 FITNESS CONSULTING INC.
Helping you make Healthy Habits a Lifestyle
(714) 261-2639

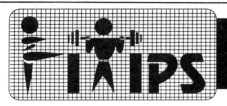

FITIPS
October 1997

Go Elastic!!

One of the most challenging things about an exercise program is fitting it into our schedule. Wouldn't it be great if we could exercise while we are commuting back and forth to work??

Well, we haven't figured out how to install an exercise bike in your front seat, but we do have an idea for doing your resistance training anytme - anywhere.

Elastic Bands!!

They are terrific!! Just pull one out of your purse or brief-case and start pulling!

And they are cheap!! If you pay more than $15 for an elastic band you got "took".

Look at the neat things you can do:

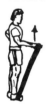

Biceps
Hold one end of the band, palm up, in your left hand, with the band's other end securely under the arch of your left foot. Start with your arm extended **without locking your elbow** and slowly pull up. Lower **slowly**, and repeat. Change sides.

Triceps
Fold a towel lengthwise and wrap around your neck. Place your band on top of the towel. Holding an end in each hand, elbows at a right angle, palms facing inward, slowly pull down. Release slowly, and repeat.

Shoulder
Tie the band to a stationary object about waist height.

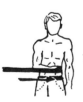

(How about a middle file drawer??) Stand with your shoulder about a foot from the file cabinet, with your elbow next to your side at a right angle.

Keeping your elbow at your side, slowly move the band across your body. Return slowly. Then pull with the other arm from the same position. Change sides.

Back
Sit on the floor with your legs extended, soft knees. Holding one end of the band in each hand, place the middle across the arches of your feet. Starting with your arms extended (don't lock your elbows!), keeping your back straight and your shoulders down, slowly pull back your elbows, squeezing together your shoulder blades. Hold a few seconds, release, and repeat.

Hamstrings & Bum
Tie band ends together, and place under one foot and around the other ankle. Standing straight, knees soft, using a wall for support, slowly lift your back leg against the tension. Lower slowly and repeat.

Outer Thigh
Keeping the band around your ankles, using a chair for support, slowly life your leg sideways. Slowly release and repeat. Change sides.

Inner Thigh
Untie your band, pulling it through the bottom file drawer handle, and re-tie. With your right shoulder toward the cabinet, place your right foot in the loop, pulling across your body. Slowly release and repeat. Turn around and change legs.

The pull and release on all these exercises is done slowly. Never let the band "snap" back.

See you at the file cabinet!

 FITNESS
CONSULTING
INC.
Since 1985
Helping you make Healthy Habits a Lifestyle
(714) 261-2639

Safety Tips

To avoid "getting slapped", always remember the following:

1. Wrap the band securely around your hand so it won't slip.
2. When fastening the band to a stationary object, make sure it's stationary!! i.e. When using a door knob, make sure the door won't open.
3. Tie the band around your foot rather than just standing on it.
4. When tying a band into a knot, make sure it is secure.

Step #4

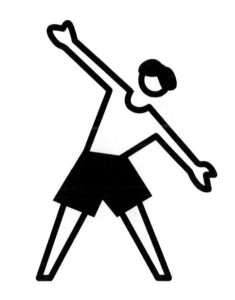

Stretching

Stretching is the number one most convenient, least time consuming activity you can do that gives you the greatest return on investment.

If you follow no other recommendations from this book except this one, you will feel much better.

Why Stretch?

Two primary benefits:

1. Lowers your risk of injury.

OK, so you're not going out to play football or rugby, why would you worry about getting injured?

American business spends over $181 billion per year paying for employee injuries on and off the job. (Studies show most are NOT rugby related...) People get injured at work every day. And it's not fun for anyone. Stretch in the morning and throughout the day and you will dramatically lower your risk of getting hurt.

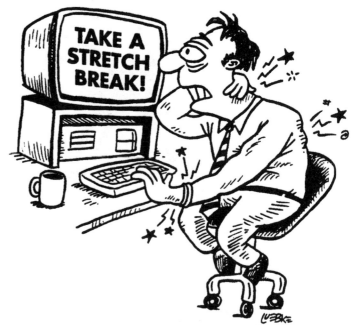

"But", you say, "I sit at my desk all day. I am not going to get hurt."

All the more reason to stretch.

Today's sedentary work style is a significant cause of injuries. We sit all day - get stiff and sore - then we bend down to pull a cord from an electrical socket and ...

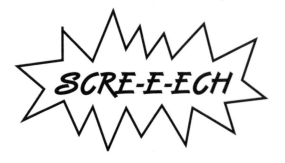

there goes the back.

Take a wild stab at which department in a large California department store has the greatest number of injuries?

Shipping/Warehouse, right?

Wrong.

Shoes?

Nope.

Aah hah! The Administrative staff!

Wrong again.

Cosmetics.

The women are generally wearing high heals (women's curse...), they are working in a confined space, and they bend down in a contorted manner to reach a lipstick below the counter and...

there it goes. Back sprain.

But you can experience these important benefits by taking moments* (honestly...<u>moments</u>) throughout the day to stretch.

*moment: an instant; a very short space of time

The second profound advantage to stretching is Stress Management!

All day long we pound away at our "to do" list - going, going, going - with barely enough time to breathe. By day's end we are often tired and frustrated, with our shoulders up to our ear lobes with tension.

Let it go!

Take time throughout the day to get rid of the stress,
bit by bit.

Even 30 seconds of rolling your shoulders will make you feel better.

Tilting your head from side to side relaxes your neck muscles.

It feels good!

And releases tension.

And only takes a moment...

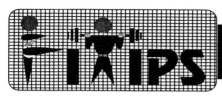

FITIPS
March 1995

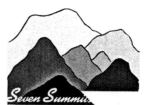

Seven Summits
A Journey for the venturesome of spirit.

Stress Relief in Minutes!

Are your neck and shoulders sore at the end of the day? Do you feel pain in your wrists? Are you tired of feeling **tired and achey**?

Well, you deserve a break today. Or maybe two or three breaks. And during those breaks, your body would love to STRETCH.

Stretching provides maximum benefits with a minimal time commitment. And the greatest benefit is its convenience. It requires no special equipment. It takes less than a minute. And you can do it anywhere. So why don't we??

Not only will regular stretching release tension and stress, it will make you much less susceptible to injury. Injury and pain are **no fun!** And consistent stretching is the key to prevention.

Following are some basic stretches, and ideas for incorporating them into your day:

Head Tilt
Tilt your head from side, to front, to side, in twenty second intervals. DO NOT TILT YOUR HEAD BACKWARDS! You may simultaniously bring alternate arm behind you and pull.

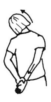

Shoulder Shrug
Lift your shoulders to your ears for 10 seconds, then let them drop.

Arm Cross Chest
Extend one arm out, across your chest. With your alternate arm, pull it toward you at the elbow.

Over the Head Press
Interlace your fingers, palms up, over your head.

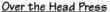

Front Press
Clasp your fingers and press with palms outward.

Seven Summits Challenge:
Take time to stretch 20 times this month

Calf Stretch
Place one foot behind the other. Press the knee of your back foot toward the floor, keeping the heel on the floor.

Tricep/Shoulder Pull
Place the palm of one hand in the middle of your back. With the other hand, pull down at the elbow.

Some stretching reminders:

- Stretching should feel relaxing. If you are feeling pain, you have gone too far.

- Stretching is a **process**. Your flexibility will gradually increase over time. Enjoy the changes.

- Don't forget to **breathe** when you stretch. Your muscles need that oxygen, so deep breathing will facilitate your stretching.

- Hold each stretch 20-30 seconds.

So when are we ever going to find time for all these stretches?!?
Following are some perfect opportunities:
- while in your car waiting at stoplights (or traffic...[grumble, grumble,...])
- at your desk
- standing at the copy machine
- standing in line at the grocery
- standing in line at the bank
- standing in line...
- while waiting for an elevator
- in the "reading room"
- while waiting for an appointment
- at break time
- waiting for the bus or carpool
- in the dentist's office (a perfect time to de-stress!)

FITNESS CONSULTING INC. *Helping you make Healthy Habits a Lifestyle*
(714) 261-2639   (916) 444-9355

Stretching Opportunities*

Stop light strategy

Here you are, sitting at a stop light...again. The 12th in a series of blocks. Is the City aware that these lights are <u>perfectly synchronized</u>? That the minute my light turns green, the next one immediately turns yellow!! Don't they know we have better things to do than sit at stop lights!

So, stretch! Nod your head to the right...feel the cartilage crunch?...take a deep breath... now nod to the left...breathe again...feel the neck stretch and relax...

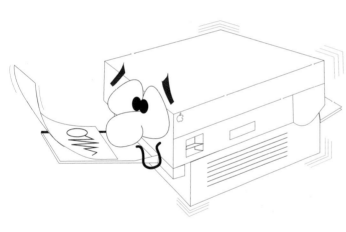

Copier's Trot

Here you are, standing at the copy machine, waiting patiently for your job to finish. Ho hum...la de da...How much longer until lunch?...

Maximize the moment! Stretch!

Is there a file cabinet nearby? Hang on to the top and bend forward, allowing your head to hang between your arms. This loosens your neck, shoulders and upper back.

No file cabinet? Then simply roll those shoulders while you wait. Forward first, then backward.

* Opportunity: A good chance for advancement or progress; a favorable or advantageous combination of circumstances; snooze, you lose.

Note: Again, Human Kinetics at www.humankinetics.com will offer a variety of books on stretching. Don't miss Bob Anderson's, appropriately entitled "Stretching".

The Office Circuit

Post different stretches at various locations throughout your office, focusing on a different body part/work area. i.e.

copy machine	=	hamstrings/quads
fax	=	arms
file cabinets	=	neck & shoulders
coffee/break room	=	back

As you move through these areas throughout the day, take a moment to do the stretches.

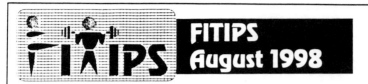
FITIPS
August 1998

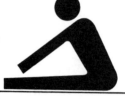

Hooked on Yoga

Life goes in cycles, so they say. And the popularity of yoga today may be proof of the pudding. This ancient Eastern discipline is finding it's niche in our harried Western culture. From health clubs to community centers, Park and Recreation and Mediation Centers, yoga is the hot ticket.

And rightly so, as even the novice Yogi will experience tremendous physical benefits.

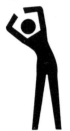
First and foremost, it it an unbeatable stretch program. We have consistently encour aged the one-minute stretch in FiTips, and will continue to endorse those miraculous moments. But there is just nothing like a solid hour of deep breathing and stretching. Aches and pains you had resigned to live with forever will disappear.

And relaxing? You can't believe how relaxing! It is alledged I have been heard snoring by the end of class! So if you are looking for a gentle way to unload some stress, yoga may be your answer. The last 8-10 minutes of every class is a final relaxation exercise. With soft music in the back ground, the instructor will talk you through a visualization meant to completely relax you. i.e. you are in the woods by a stream, sitting on a hillside under a tree listening to the birds, etc. You will truly feel like you have "been away".

Yoga is an excellent vehicle for improving circulation and therefore energy. Once you awaken from your "relaxation coma", you will feel more energetic and vital. Yoga proponents contend it will also improve your digestive and immune systems, as many of the poses,  or asanas, were developed for that purpose. And there must be something to that, because many hospitals across the country are incorporating yoga and meditation into their therapy programs.

For any who are interested, yoga can also be a spiritual discipline, which was its original intent. The word yoga is derived from the Sanskrit word yoj, meaning "to bind or attach; to concentrate one's attention on". So the purpose was to unite the practitioner's mind, body and spirit with the will of God. Many use it as an active form of meditation.

There are actually several forms of yoga, though the most commonly practiced in our Western society is Hatha Yoga. As you advance, however, you may want to investigate one of the others, such as Bhakti, Raja, or Jnana, which are more individualized for specific personality types, strengths and weaknesses.

When starting a yoga class, wear clothing that allows you freedom of movement. Cycling shorts or tights, and a t-shirt are best. Feet are bare.

Before your first class, introduce yourself to the instructor and tell him/her about any pains or injuries you need to watch. A good instructor will provide alternate versions of the difficult poses for those who are less flexible. Instructors can get certified in some places in six weeks, and others take several years, so inquire about your instructor's credentials.

Who should consider yoga?

Everyone! It's terrific for all us "aging athletes" to stretch out those aches and pains. Anyone with back, neck or shoulder pain will find it helpful. Have arthritis? Yoga will certainly help. Over 50 and a bit intimidated by the health club scene? Try yoga. Bar none, everyone can benefit. And that is one of the greatest aspects of yoga, that people of all fitness levels can work together. Every posture can be done at your own level.

<u>Remember:</u> You are there for <u>YOU</u>. Move at your own pace. Watch and enjoy your own progress. And remember, it's a *process*.

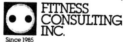
FITNESS
CONSULTING
INC.
Since 1985

Helping you make Health Habits a Lifestyle
(714) 261-2639   www.fitnessconsulting.com

Exercise

OK. Time to rethink your exercise prescription.

This time we need to consider all the components
of a well-rounded program.

Still ...

It must be <u>realistic.</u>

It must be <u>strategic</u>.
(appropriate given your goals)

It must be <u>fun</u>!

What days will you exercise? _____

What time of day will you exercise? _____

How long will each session be? _____

What will you do at each session?_____

_____

_____

_____

Have you included aerobic, stretching, and strength training?

Step #5

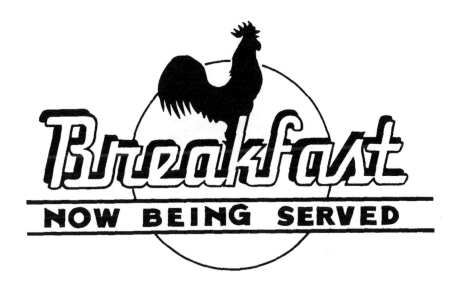

No
Meal
Skipping

Timing

Timing of your food is every bit as important as your food choices themselves.

Before we concern ourselves with <u>what</u> we are going to eat (which is a never ending process), let's start with timing...

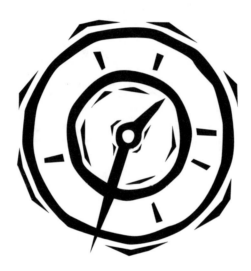

NO MEAL SKIPPING

Skipping meals is self-sabotage.

It trains your body to store fat.

It robs you of energy.

It heightens your vulnerability to making poor food choices later.

Eating regularly, every 3-4 hours, is vital*.

It stabilizes your blood sugar.

It keeps your energy consistent.

It heightens your resistance to binging.

* vital: necessary to the existence, continuance, or *well-being* of something; indispensable; essential; pretty darned important.

Timing is Everything

One of the many challenges in today's hectic world is taking time to eat. Instead of taking breaks throughout the day to refuel, we go from one meeting to another, one commitment to the next, eating nothing (except maybe a candy bar...) all day. By day's end we are ravenous, and eat anything and everything in sight.

Sound familiar?

In caring for your body, **YOU MUST EAT!** Remember, food is your friend. Your body needs fuel. Taking time to eat is taking care of you.

At the risk of sounding unromantic, consider the analogy of fuel in a car. You wouldn't try to drive your car without gas, would you? (...don't answer that...) So why do you try to "drive" your body without fuel?

Unfortunately there is no "Human A.A.A." to bail us out. And consider these negative repercussions of skipping meals:

1. It teaches your body to store fat. (Ugh!)

Any time you miss meals, your body kicks into survival mode and starts storing fat in self defense. This is its natural response in the event you are ever caught on a desert island and needed to stay alive without food. So every time you allow several hours (4-5+) to pass without "gassing up", you are telling your body to store fat. Is that really the message you want to send?

2. It robs you of energy.

Ever feel like you have run out of gas? Tired and lethargic? Headache? "Less than pleasant" mood? Well, have you ever considered maybe you ARE out of gas? When was the last time you ate? Part of America's fatigue factor is lack of fuel. Food is our "go juice", and we are constantly trying to "Go" without any juice. Skip meals and you are sure to be more tired.

3. It increases your vulnerability to poor food choices.

Back to the example above. You have gone all day without taking time to eat, and now you are home, raging hungry. What do you choose? An apple? Some veggies with a little nonfat Ranch dip? Maybe a turkey sandwich? Heck no!! Go for the chips and salsa! And don't forget the beer! You are so hungry that guess what? In no time the entire bag of chips has disappeared. Remember: The quality of your food choices seems to be indirectly correlated to your hunger factor.

The goal is to have a consistent energy level, clear mental acuity, and relaxed self control. These require regular fuel stops.

Ideally, plan to eat every 3-4 hours. That simply means incorporating a mid-morning and mid-afternoon snack into your day. Your body metabolizes smaller, more regular portions better than larger, less frequent meals. This fuel regimen will keep your blood sugar even and your energy level consistent. The digestion of the food also keeps your metabolism elevated, which actually makes you burn fat more efficiently. So bottom line is eat more often and you will lose more fat! Gotta like that!!

So what does a typical day look like? Something like this...

6:30am   Bowl of cereal with fruit and nonfat milk

9:30am   Whole wheat bagel with lowfat cream cheese

12:00   Lunch - pasta w/lean meat sauce and veggies
- beans, rice and veggies
- potato with nonfat cottage cheese
- lentil soup and brown bread

3:00pm   Piece of fruit

6:00pm   Dinner - Big salad
- Veggie omelette with egg whites
- Vegetable soup with brown bread

Exercise

Are you a breakfast skipper? Why? _____

_____

_____

Didn't your mother teach you that "Breakfast is your most important meal"?

It is, indeed, a fact.

Remember, you are starting to consider food your fuel - "something that gives nourishment or incentive" - and we awaken each day "on empty". To insure energy and vitality, we <u>must</u> refuel.

Starting each day with breakfast will also facilitate your weight management program. Remember the survival mode thing? Well, when you consistently skip breakfast, going without nourishment from 8:00pm-12noon the next day, your body will store fat in self defense.

!! Bottom Line: Eating a healthy breakfast makes you a better fat burner!

" But I'm just not hungry in the morning..."

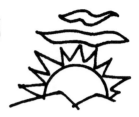

Your body naturally wants to be fed. The word breakfast, when broken down into its component parts, means "breaking the fast". Since dinner/supper the previous evening, you have been "fasting". When you awaken your body is ready for fuel. At one time it sent you "hunger pangs". In time, after you consistently ignored it, it quit sending the pangs.

This doesn't mean it no longer wants breakfast! It simply stops sending signals and goes into self defense/starvation mode - storing fat for future "fasts".

So how do you get back into the breakfast habit, when truthfully, you are <u>not</u> interested?

Start slowly.

Begin with a piece of toast.

Then go to toast and a piece of fruit.

Next try a bowl of cereal.

Before long you will notice those morning hunger pangs returning.
And you will <u>want</u> to take time for some breakfast.
Because you have noticed you feel better when you do...

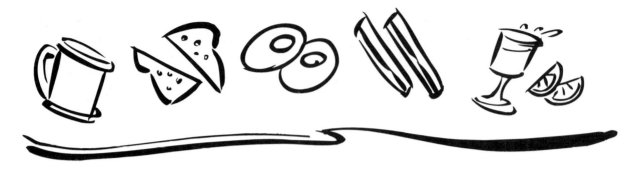

Breakfast Boosters*

QUICKIES:

Bagel** with: nonfat/lowfat cream cheese
: <u>light</u> peanut butter*** and honey
: jam, man.
: lite cream cheese, tomato & cucumber
: nonfat cottage cheese & cinnamon

Can't beat cereal.

oatmeal
cheerios
shredded wheat
grape nuts
all bran

one at a time,
or mix 'em up!

with 1C nonfat milk and fruit.

* Booster: a person or thing that elevates, increases or raises, especially energy or enthusiasm; a pick-em-up.

** Whole wheat bagels have more fiber than those made with plain white flour. And store bought bagels have come a long way! Have you tried the new whole wheats?

***Peanut butter is 82% fat. It is mostly unsaturated, however, so it will never clog your arteries. But remember light means "thinly spread on the bread". You're not trying to set a brick.

Fabulous French Toast!

<u>Mix:</u> 3 egg whites
1 whole egg
1/8C nonfat milk
cinnamon
nutmeg (optional)

Dip and brown in non-stick
skillet, and/or use cooking spray.

<u>Top with:</u> vanilla yogurt
hot apple sauce
fresh fruit
light syrup

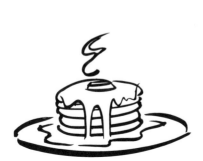

Love those **Buckwheats!**

Follow the directions on good ol'
Aunt Jemima's Buckwheat Pancake mix
with a few minor changes.
· Use nonfat milk,
· two egg whites/egg and
· replace oil with apple sauce.
· See toppings above.

Bacon, anyone?

Don't feel like you've gotta go without.
Try any of the turkey bacon alternatives.

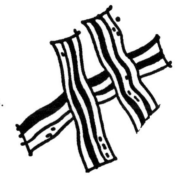

Egg White Omelette

Throw in one whole egg, 3-4 whites, and all the veggies that aren't yet "growing" in your refrigerator.

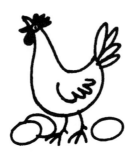

- onions
- green and red peppers
- broccoli (sorry, George...)
- zucchini
- spinach**

** Just like ordering a pizza!

Unfried Potatoes

Dice potato(es) into small pieces, place them in a plastic bag, and nuke them approximately 8-10 minutes. Saute veggies (onion, green pepper, mushrooms) in a frying pan with a tad* bit of olive oil. Add potatoes, and spice with a little cajun.

* tad: a skosh, a pinch; a little. *ant:* veggies taking a swim

Step #6

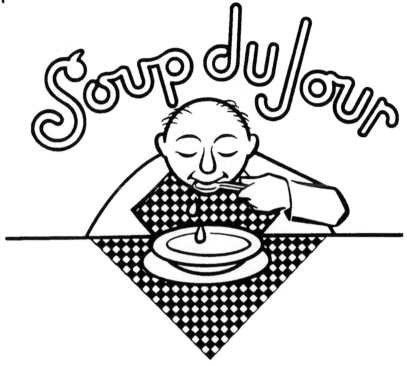

Eat

Top Heavy

Generally speaking we are not going to spend a lot of time in this program counting calories. If you are choosing the right foods, at the right times, you really need not bother worrying about specific calorie count.

But therein lie two key qualifiers!

The right foods, which we will discuss in later chapters,

at the right times!

Remember you are trying to think of your food as **fuel** - <u>nourishment for your body</u>. So it should be obvious that it makes sense to "gas up before the trip!"

Your "trip", or primary energy expenditure, is the active part of your day. You burn limited calories at night while reading a book or watching TV. And you expend even less while you are sleeping.

SO WHY IS <u>DINNER</u> SO OFTEN
OUR <u>BIGGEST</u> MEAL OF THE DAY?

That's like gassing up after reaching your destination!

Oh sure, your body saves it for tomorrow's fuel. Some is stored as glycogen or glucose. But that bowl of ice cream gets stored as <u>fat</u>! So the challenge is to take in calories as you will use them, typically meaning

Eat Top Heavy.

Your largest meals should be breakfast and lunch, with dinner being lighter.*

---

*   For all you shift workers, interpret "breakfast" as your first meal, lunch your second meal, etc. regardless of what time your day starts.

Let's take a look at how you are doing. Following is a Calorie Flow Chart. Identify the foods you eat at each meal, and approximate their calories. Then **bracket on center** the count on the designated line, with every hash mark representing 100 calories*. (If you are unsure about calories, approximate, or read your labels!)

Calorie Flow Chart

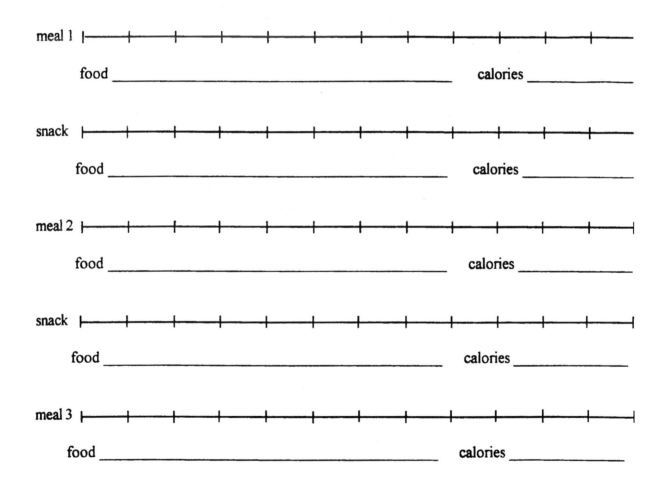

meal 1

food _____ calories _____

snack

food _____ calories _____

meal 2

food _____ calories _____

snack

food _____ calories _____

meal 3

food _____ calories _____

*   For the Big Boys who are BIG eaters, have each mark represent 200 calories.

Sample Calorie Flow Chart

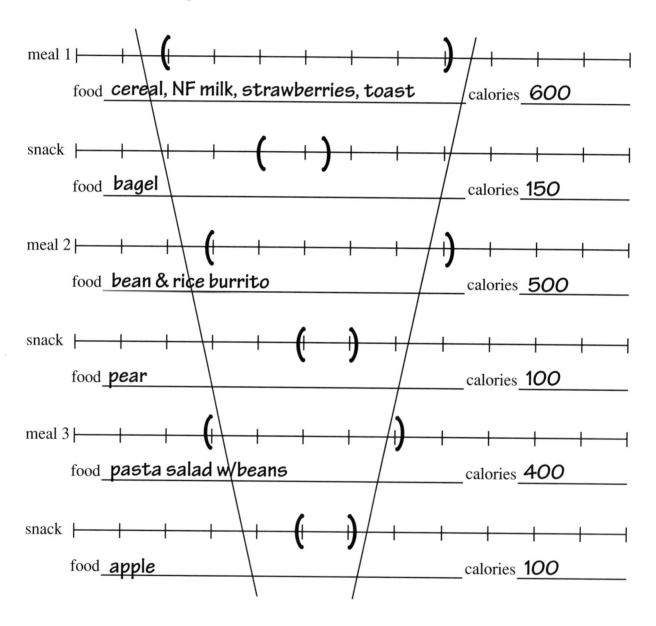

meal 1

food cereal, NF milk, strawberries, toast   calories 600

snack

food bagel   calories 150

meal 2

food bean & rice burrito   calories 500

snack

food pear   calories 100

meal 3

food pasta salad w/beans   calories 400

snack

food apple   calories 100

The goal is to create an upside down triangle. Now that may mean meals that gradually decrease in size throughout the day, or the first two or three similar in size with dinner being smaller. But you definitely need to taper at the bottom!

Now let's look at Barry's Calorie Flow Chart:

Calorie Flow Chart

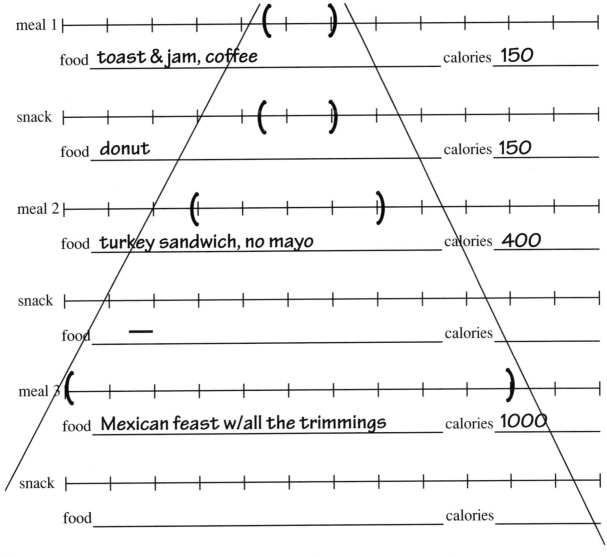

meal 1
food __toast & jam, coffee__ calories __150__

snack
food __donut__ calories __150__

meal 2
food __turkey sandwich, no mayo__ calories __400__

snack
food __—__ calories __

meal 3
food __Mexican feast w/all the trimmings__ calories __1000__

snack
food __ calories __

His trangle ain't upside down!

As Easy as Your Morning Coffee

Calorie Flow Chart

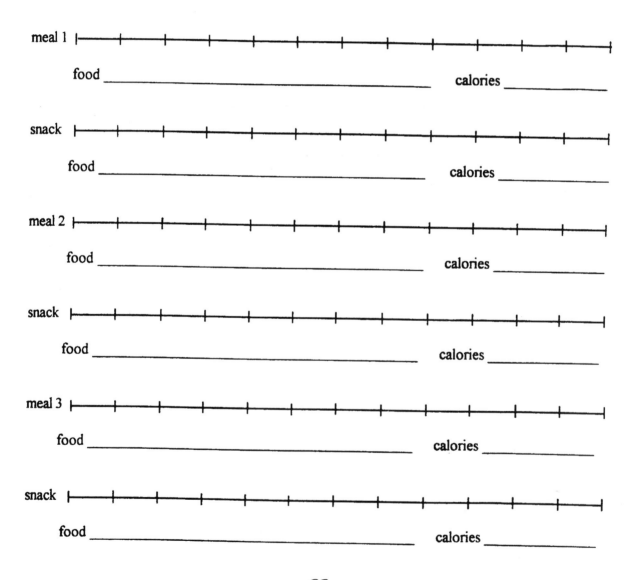

meal 1 |————————————————————————|

food _____ calories _____

snack |————————————————————————|

food _____ calories _____

meal 2 |————————————————————————|

food _____ calories _____

snack |————————————————————————|

food _____ calories _____

meal 3 |————————————————————————|

food _____ calories _____

snack |————————————————————————|

food _____ calories _____

Eating "upside down" may prove to be challenging. Our culture is no longer geared this way. The days of a big family breakfast, dinner mid-day, with supper (smaller) in the evening are gone.

Many today claim to be "too busy" for both breakfast and lunch, so guess who pigs out at dinner?

Even restaurants serve us backwards. Lunch entrees are typically smaller than dinner. Or some offer "half orders" at lunch. It is lunchtime when we should be eating!!

Conversely, I recently dined at a small establishment offering southwestern cuisine. A friend and I wanted to split a dinner entree and they wanted to charge us $1.50 for the extra plate!

Exercise

Make enough Calorie Flow Charts for the entire week and graph your meals.

How to Lighten Up

One of the challenges of lightening up dinner is understanding <u>how</u>. Big dinners are simply a habit. Following are some **Dinner Lite** ideas.

<u>Salad Grandioso</u>

In a big bowl, throw in all the colors of the harvest - greens, yellows, reds, oranges. Top it with one of the following:

- · kidney beans
- · potato
- · tuna salad w/ NF mayo
- · nonfat cottage cheese
- · pieces of chicken/fish

  Then use you favorite lowfat/nonfat dressing.

<u>Soup and Brown Bread</u> - Hearty, healthy, yummy. But steer clear of cream soups!

<u>Shish-K-Bobs</u> - Fill your skewers with luscious veggies and chunks of fish. Serve with rice.

<u>Mays Heart Special</u>* - Black beans, brown rice, lotsa veggies and killer salsa.

*   from The Village Farmer, Santa Ana, CA

Don't Destroy the Moment

"But", some of you are saying, "the evening meal is the one time of day our family can have quality time together. It just won't be the same over carrots and celery!"

Remember, I am <u>not</u> suggesting you not eat!   I am simply reminding you to eat light.

And the family gathering can be enhanced with healthy fare. You are nurturing and celebrating your family and their health by making wise food choices. The ambiance need not be ruined!

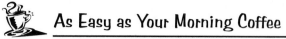

Step #7

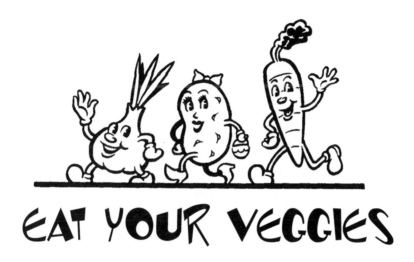

EAT YOUR VEGGIES

5-a-Day

5-a-Day

Since we were kids we have been prodded, "Eat your vegetables!", usually followed by, "They're good for you."

"They're good for you." What does that mean?

Well, recent studies are providing answers to that question in greater and greater depth. Vegetables are beginning to rival exercise in their number of significant benefits. Let's take a look...

The Inside Scoop

Ever stop to consider all the activity going on in your body at any given time? Talk about a hap'nin' place! Your internal action makes Grand Central Station look calm!

Consider, for example, your cell's metabolism of food and oxygen. During that process, particles called "free radicals" are released. They are called free radicals because they are short one electron, and are trolling for their compatible "spark". Liken them to single humans. In search of "electricity" and bonding, they often find themselves with the "unperfect" match that leads to trouble. And so it is with free radicals. Free radicals often react with otherwise healthy cells, causing structural damage and disease. Studies reveal that stress, cigarette smoke, and radiation speed the negative effects of free radical activity.

Enter "The Good Guys". Antioxydants, found in fruits and vegetables, serve as "escorts" to the free radicals. They "get them off the street" so to speak. Bonding with the free radicals makes them less reactive, reducing cell damage, specifically heart disease and cancer.

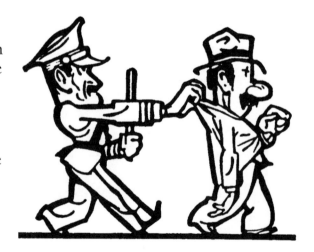

Some antioxydants are manufactured by the cells themselves, but three Superstars, Vitamins C and E, and beta carotene, are plentiful in fruits and vegetables.

Carrots in a Pill

Typical American "Can-I-get-it-in-a-pill?" mentality, the mid '90's saw the promotion of over-the-counter antioxydants. Along with the enlightenment about antioxydants came the commercialism of supplements. Consumers flocked to markets and health food stores buying their beta carotene. Why stop for a salad when I can pop a pill?

Unfortunately, you just can't fool Mother Nature. Recent studies indicate that antioxydants via supplements have NOT proven effective in preventing cancer, and in some cases, even exacerbated the condition.

Oooopps. Grandma was right.
Eat your vegetables.

Ok, now that we have confirmed with high-powered studies and big words that Grandma's plea to "Eat your vegetables!" was sage advice, how do we do it? Does a salad from McDonalds with iceberg lettuce, a few carrot scrapings and a cherry tomato do it for you?

Following are some ideas that would make Grandma proud...

- Put tomato, sprouts, grated carrot and spinach on sandwiches (iceberg lettuce has 1254 IU Vitamin A per 1/2 C; spinach has 2230!)

- Put fruit on your morning cereal. (Of course you are eating breakfast now, aren't you?) Enjoy the fruits of the season.

- Eat fruit for a snack and you're 2/5.

- Load your soups, pasta salads and sauces with veggies.

- Cut up cucumbers, carrots, broccoli and cauliflower on Sunday evening for snacking throughout the week. Have nonfat Ranch or Blue Cheese salad dressing on hand for dip.

- Put veggies in your egg white omelettes. Then top with salsa. MMMmmmmmm....!

- Buy the prepared Salad Fixin's for easier salad preparation. (Get the spinach and/or mixed greens. Steer clear of generic iceberg.)

- Baby carrots, snow peas, sweet peas and green beans are easy snacks. Just rinse and munch!

- Cut up an orange for your lunch box. If you take it whole, chances are you won't eat it.

- Make cole slaw with apples and raisins, using nonfat coleslaw dressing. (They'll never know it's nonfat at the potluck...)

- When dining out, eat veggie soup instead of the traditional iceberg lettuce salad.

- Try a bagel with nonfat or lowfat cream cheese, topped with a tomato slice and a hint of fresh basil.

- How about a peanut butter and banana or peanut butter and apple sandwich? Remember, go light on the pb.

- Steamed veggies over rice, dressed with seasoned rice vinegar is a winner dinner.

- Fresh salsa, made with tomatoes, onions, peppers, and cilantro makes a great potato topping.

- Put grapes, blueberries, or raspberries in the freezer for a healthy sweet treat.

As you begin increasing your veggie intake, remember to go for a variety of colors - reds, yellows, greens, oranges - to insure a variety of nutrients.

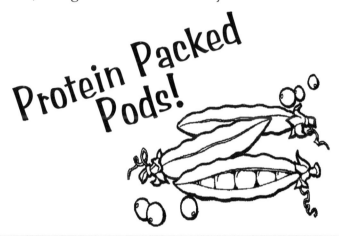

Peas...Did You Know?...

You may have not spent much time contemplating the pea. But did you know that 2/3C. of peas has 6 gm. of protein, more than a whole egg or a tsp. of peanut butter? And furthermore, are you aware that peas have been with us for centuries? That archealogists found dried peas in the Egyptian tombs? But honestly, my fascination with peas is not about historical connection. It's because **they're easy**! Buy them frozen and they look, taste, and retain the nutrients of fresh. But there's no pod popping. No chopping like carrots. No shredding like lettuce and spinach. You don't even have to wash them! Just throw them in salads, casseroles (big in the Midwest, especially at church potlucks...) soups, chili, pasta sauce, milkshakes, (well, maybe not...) and insta-protein.

Oh, and did I mention there's as much
vitamin C in 3/4 C. peas as an orange?!

Step #8

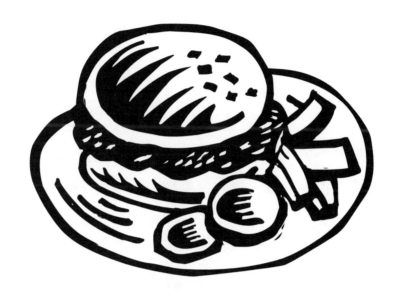

Say "NO" to FAT!

The Food Pyramid

In 1994 the Food and Drug Administration introduced the food pyramid to assist us in making our daily food choices. And believe it or not, this time your tax dollars went toward a very valuable program. On many food labels you will see the pyramid below.

The message is straightforward:

The bottom of your pyramid, or the basis of all your meals, should be complex carbohydrates; breads, cereals, grains, potatoes, and pasta. The recommended number of servings is 6-11 per day.

Why?

Because carbohydrates are the most easily converted to glucose which is what your body uses for fuel. They are premium gasoline. And since most of what we eat is utilized as energy, carbos are the way to go.

To get the benefits of fiber you want to eat mostly whole grains. And remember: Variety is the spice of life!

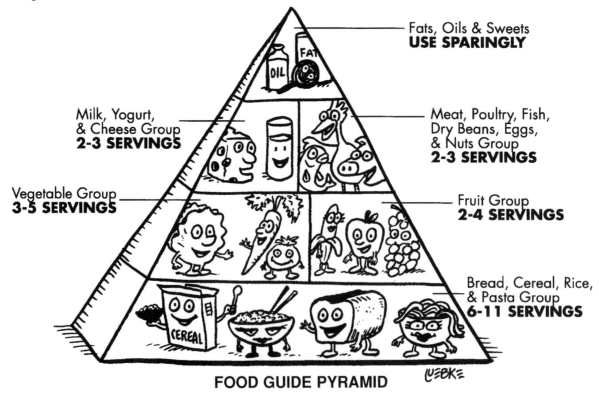

FOOD GUIDE PYRAMID

A True Story

A few years ago I had the opportunity to work with a very talented high school athlete. She was working diligently to lower her body fat, so she started reducing her dietary fat intake, focusing more on complex carbohydrates and moderate protein.

At one of our consultations I asked her to describe a typical day's food choices.

"I normally have a bagel for breakfast, with a little light cream cheese."

OK. Any mid-morning snacks?

"I usually have another bagel."

Hmmmmm... "OK, and tell me about lunch."

"Well, there's a bagel place across the street from my school, so I usually have a turkey bagel sandwich."

AAaaaahhh!

Just because bagels have been deemed "good for us" doesn't mean we should consume them breakfast, lunch and dinner! Because they are easily accessible and extremely durable, I have seen people use bagels as their food staple. Remember, the 6-11 servings of complex carbohydrates should be a <u>variety</u> of grains and cereals.

" Man (not woman) does not live by bagels alone!"

And remember, when you do grab a bagel, go for the whole wheat or multi grain.

"Second Floor..."

The second level on your pyramid is the Fruits and Vegetable Department. We have already discussed their many benefits. The pyramid simply confirms their value in the food chain. And in fact, it ups the ante from "5-a-day" to 3-5 veggies and 2-4 fruits. So the 5-a-day mix is a minimum.

"Proteins"

Proteins are a critical nutritional ingredient. They are the guys who repair, rebuild and maintain your tissue and fluid systems. So moderate protein is a must.

Americans, however, have a tendency to overshop in the Protein Department. We <u>love</u> our meat and cheese! Bacon or sausage for breakfast, hamburgers or turkey sandwiches for lunch, and fish, chicken or steak for dinner. There also have been several high protein diets that have lured people in by promising rapid weight loss. **High protein diets are extremely hard on your liver and kidneys!** The weight loss is a result of <u>water</u> loss as your body works diligently to rid itself of the excess nitrogen resulting from the protein breakdown. It is not a healthy nor permanent weight loss solution.

Remember, protein is the side show at every meal, NOT the main attraction! Fruits and veggies, pasta, rice and potatoes should be in the limelight, especially early in the day.

So next time you sit down to a meal, look at your plate. What food(s) are stealing the show? The big hunk of beef? or the platter of noodles?

Consider the Asian cuisines, loaded with rice and veggies, with a bit of chicken, fish or beef.

And Viva Italiano! with lotsa veggies and noodles and a complementary meatball.

A Little Protein in Every Bite

As you make your meal and snack choices, consider the protein complement concept. Studies show that our bodies prefer a little protein at every meal. So think about the following:

INSTEAD OF...	HAVE...
plain bagel	a bagel with light cream cheese
toast and butter	toast with light peanut butter
baked potato with sour cream	baked potato with cottage cheese
rice and veggies	beans, rice and veggies (or chopped egg whites)
an all veggie salad	beans, cottage cheese or egg whites with your greens (and yellows, and reds, and...)

"Fourth Floor. Going Down."

You may have noticed that all the "good stuff", donuts, pastries, french fries, are at the peak of the pyramid. Great view from the top, but restricted to the "chosen few". Unless you have been hiding under a rock over the past decade plus, you are aware of the physical hazards of fats, especially animal and/or saturated fats. But let's review the basics:

1. Fats make you fat.

A gram of a carbohydrate or protein are 4 calories. A gram of fat is 9.

So pound for pound (or gram by gram...) you get nearly 2 1/2 times the number of calories when you eat fat as when you choose carbos or proteins.

Example:

Baked potato	145 calories	.2gm fat
Sour cream (2T)	62 calories	6gm fat

The sour cream adds 43% more calories, 88% of which are FAT!

Now, add 1/2C. (4 times more!) of nonfat cottage cheese and you get <u>no</u> fat, and 14 grams of protein! (vs. 1gm. protein in the 2T. sour cream).

* See "How to Calculate % Calories from Fat"

2. Fats make you sleepy.

Understand that when you eat fatty foods, the fat gets into the blood and makes your red blood cells stick together, so your blood gets "thicker". As a result, it's flow through your system slows, reducing the amount of oxygen to your heart, brain, muscles, etc. (see graphic next page)

Bottom line: You feel sleepy.

3. Fats elevate your blood pressure.

Let's review our notes from "Basic Plumbing 101". Your arteries are your pipes.

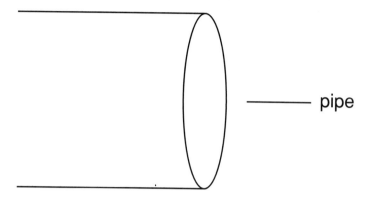 pipe

As the red blood cells scurry through your "pipes", they create a bit of pressure.

This is normal.

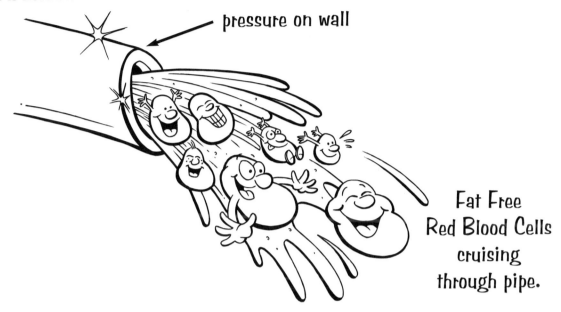

pressure on wall

Fat Free
Red Blood Cells
cruising
through pipe.

What do you suppose happens to that pressure when the fluid in your pipes turns from water-like to <u>sludge</u> because you have chosen to eat something full of fat?

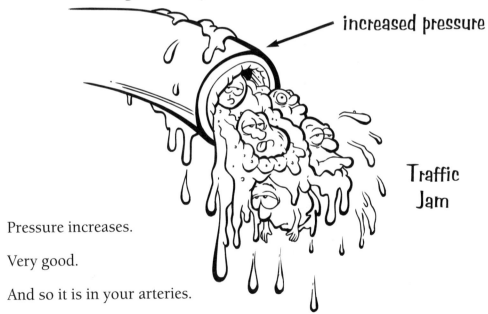

increased pressure

Traffic
Jam

Pressure increases.

Very good.

And so it is in your arteries.

Blood changes from happy, free-floating, cruise-thru-your-arteries red blood cells to stuck-together, fat-filled sludge, so pressure in your "pipes" increases, possibly dangerously.

4. Fat can kill you.

Back to the plumbing analogy. For 30, 40, 50, maybe even 60 or more years you have been eating fat. Saturated fat. In your arteries fat. Day after day that sludge has been flowing through your pipes.

Take a wild stab at what the inside of your pipes look like.

Yep.

Cruddy.

Much of that fat never made it through the system. It attached to the wall of your pipe and has been stuck there for years. And once some fat is stuck there, more fat gets stuck there. Fat attracts fat. Doctors call it plaque.

So now let's look at your pipe from this angle:

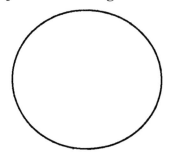

The above is a baby's artery, before her first Big Mac.

Below is the artery of a 21 year old American boy.

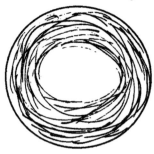

When autopsies were done on the casualties from both the Korean and Vietnam wars, many of the boys arteries were already over 50% obstructed.

They were the beginning of the fast-food generations.

Exercise

So what do you think your arteries look like??

How often do you eat:

butter
sour cream
cheese
fried foods
red meats
mayo
ice cream
eggs

Fill the "artery" below, speculating on the obstruction in your own.

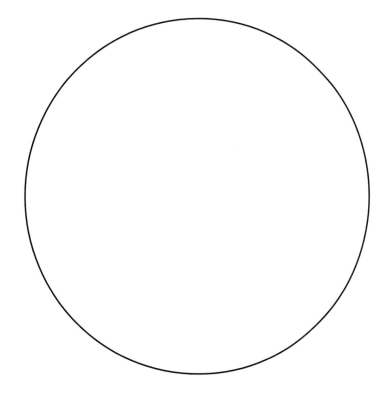

All Fats are **NOT** Created Equal

Save the Cows!

All fats do not clog your arteries.

Saturated fats - primarily animal fats - ultimately land in your arteries and cause heart disease and stroke.

Most vegetable fats do not.

The key is how <u>solid</u> the fat is at room temperature. Consider the fat on a t-bone steak. At room temperature, it's still solid. Whereas vegetable oil is fluid at room temperature. So it will stay fluid in your arteries.

So put a little* peanut butter on your morning toast and you need not concern yourself about a heart attack. (Peanut <u>oil</u> is fluid at room temperature.) Or live on the edge and choose butter.

Pile that baked potato high with nonfat cottage cheese and "no worries". Go for sour cream and your arteries get clogged.

And vinegar and oil salad dressing beats blue cheese unless the cheese is low fat.

So your challenge is to find lightened versions of your favorite foods.

And they are <u>everywhere</u>.

I cannot think of a food that is naturally high in fat that is <u>not</u> offered today in a lower fat version. Lowfat/Nonfat Cheese. Lowfat/Nonfat Ice cream. Egg beaters. Leaner cuts of beef. Nonfat salad dressings. Lowfat and nonfat mayo, sour cream and cream cheese. Even nonfat croutons and potato chips!

And lightened foods have come a l-o-n-g way! In the mid 80's we only had a few salad dressing choices, and all were pretty pathetic. They validated the complaint that healthy foods taste terrible. But today, there are more brands and "flavors" of nonfat salad dressings than ever before. And they taste great!! If you can't find one you like, you're really not trying!

*   *Little: A small amount; a smidge; less than you usually do and would like*

So let's review the list of foods high in saturated fats:

- cheese
- eggs
- whole milk
- good old fashioned ice cream
- sour cream
- mayo
- butter
- margarine (see next page)
- red meats
- shellfish
- some fried foods
- lard (traditional tortillas...)

How to Calculate the percentage of fat in your foods...

So how do you know the percentage of fat in any given food?

Read your labels, and get out your calculator.

There's just one number you need to remember:

A gram of fat is 9 calories.

Knowing that, you can calculate the percentage of fat calories in any given food.

Here's the basic formula:

grams of fat/serving (from the label)
x 9 calories/gram

calories from fat
÷ total calories (from the label)

% of calories from fat

So let's look at 2% milk:

Each serving has 5 grams of fat and is 140 calories.

So...

5 grams
x 9 calories/gram

45 calories from fat
÷ 140 total calories

.32 or 32% fat

What's "Cholesterol"?

Cholesterol is a substance both manufactured in your liver and found in animal food products. It is part of the cause of the artery clogging.

There are two types of cholesterol. HDL, or high density lipoprotein, helps to keep your arteries clear. It is manufactured by your liver, and is increased with regular aerobic exercise. LDL, or low density lipoprotein, exacerbates the clogging, and increases when you eat foods from animal sources. To differentiate the two, remember "H" is for "happy" or "healthy".

So if the food I eat doesn't have cholesterol, am I home free?

Well, no. You see there is a process utilized by food manufacturers called "hydrogenization". You will see on the food labels of chips, cookies, crackers, "partially hydrogenated vegetable oil".

RED FLAG

The process of hydrogenation is actually partially <u>solidifying</u> (that "s" word...) the oil, making it look and act more like a saturated fat. They are called transfats. So good ol' vegetable oil that in its natural state would never hang around your arteries, <u>does</u> after it has been hydrogenated. Thank you food manufacturers!

NOTE: Margarine is made with hydrogenated oils, so it is really no better for you than butter.

Why do they do that?

Two reasons:

1. Hydrogenization increases the shelf life of foods, and

2. Hydrogenization allows the temperature of the oil to remain stable during the frying process, which assures consistency of taste. You <u>always</u> want your fritos to taste like fritos, don't you?

What is Hypertension and why is it bad?

Blood pressure is the pressure on your arterial walls. Normal is 120/80. The top number is called "systolic" and is the pressure in your "pipes" just as your heart is beating. It will fluctuate often throughout any given day. Stress, excitement, fear, or physical activity increase systolic blood pressure. The lower number, or diastolic, is the pressure in your arteries **between beats.**

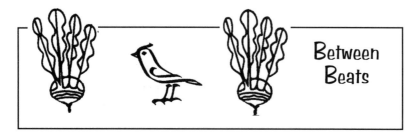

You have pressure in your arteries between heart beats, you got problems, buddy. So what can cause hypertension?

1. Stress - When you are stressed, your arteries contract. (Whats up with that!?) So about the time your whole body is screaming for more oxygen, your arteries shut down. This increases blood pressure.

2. High Fat Diet - Remember the sludge story? Eat fat - blood turns to sludge - pressure in the pipes increases.

3. Obstruction - If your pipes are full of goo* as a result of long-term consumption of saturated fats, the size of your "passageways" are reduced. Reduce the pipe size and try to process "mud" through them, and pressure increases.

* *goo: sludge, gook**, crud, schmultz, yucky stuff*

** *In Random House' dictionary (admittedly their 1975 Edition - I don't throw things away...) gook is listed just before* **goon***, defined as "a stupid person", and soon after* **goof***, "a foolish or stupid person". A coincidence?*

Did Mama lie?

Dairy Do's and Don'ts

Since we were kids we have been taught to "drink your milk". (Alas, another "it's good for you...") And today we know whole milk is loaded with saturated fat that ultimately lands in our arteries and causes heart disease and stroke.

Did Mama lie?

No. (Whew! Had a trust issue going on there...)

Some components of dairy products are good for you. They are loaded with calcium (for strong bones and teeth...) as well as Vitamin D, riboflavin and high quality protein. A cup of milk provides about 15-20% of an adult's daily protein requirement, 25% of our recommended Vitamin D, and 25-38% calcium RDA.

So Milk IS good for you!

Unfortunately, whole and even 2% milk are also loaded with saturated, clog-your-arteries fat. In fact, 48% of the calories in whole milk come from fat. Let's calculate:

$$1C \text{ whole milk}$$
$$150 \text{ calories}$$
$$8 \text{ gm fat}$$

$$8gm \times 9 \text{ cal/gm} = 72 \text{ calories}$$
$$72 \div 150 = 48\% \text{ fat!}$$

So nearly half the calories you are consuming come from fat!

Now the good news is 1% or nonfat milk provides you all the same nutrients (sometimes even higher!) without all the fat!

Check out Table 3.

Did You Know . . .

Most nondairy creamers have as many calories as light cream and contain coconut oil, which is even more saturated than butterfat.

Berkeley Wellness
Encyclopedia

Milk: The Real Scoop

	Calcium	Protein	Fat
Whole*	291mg	8 gm	8
2%	297mg	10 gm	5
1%	300mg	11 gm	2.5
Skim	302mg	9 gm	0
* 1Cup			

Table 3

So the challenge is to slowly** transition from fat-filled whole milk
to nutrient rich 1% or skim milk.

Do it over night and you'll be hating life.
Go from drinking whole milk to skim in one step and you'll feel like
you are drinking spoiled water.

Transition slowly, "one small milk step" at a time,
and each one will feel much easier.

** *Slowly: taking a long time; no rush; "Hakuna Matata!".*

Dairy Diary

How often are you eating any of the following?

	Nonfat	Lowfat	Whole
Cheese			
Yogurt			
Milk			
Eggs*			
Ice Cream**			

* Egg whites would be considered nonfat. One whole egg with extra whites would be considered lowfat. Whole eggs would be whole.

** Ice cream should only be used occasionally as a dairy source, as even lowfat and nonfat ice creams are loaded with sugar.

Copy chart and complete daily.
Ultimately strive for 2-3 servings/day
from the nonfat/lowfat side.

The Bottom Line
on
FAT

The bottom line on fat is we <u>can</u> eat some, but we want to keep within a "budget". (Don't you <u>hate</u> that!) Men should eat no more than 50gms/day. Women should stay within 40gms.

So becoming a diligent label reader of the foods you choose is a must. You must note the number of grams of fat per serving in that item, then be <u>realistic</u> about the number of servings you consume. See the following FiTips on Label Reading and Serving Sizes. And just like a checkbook, you need to keep a daily tally to be sure you don't go "over budget". So I recommend you keep a FAT REGISTER, accounting for the fat grams you consume throughout the day. Men start with a daily balance of 50. Women 40. And you will "debit" your account for every food you eat that contains fat. And remember, NO OVERDRAFTS!

Oh, and by the way. You can't transfer one day's "savings" into the next day.

<u>Sample</u>

Date	Food	Fat Debit (-)	Exercise Credit (+)	Balance (50)/ 40
9/1	cereal w/ 1C 2% milk	8		42
"	pastry	6		36
"	turkey sand w/ cheese & mayo	8		28
"	Snickers bar	14		14
"	pasta w/ meatballs salad w/LF dressing	16		<2> (Ooopps...)
"	30 extra minutes on bike		5	3

FiTips
May
1994

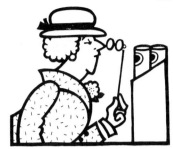

The good news is, beginning this month, the FDA has established guidelines for food labels that should ultimately make it easier to make healthy food choices. The bad news is, in the short term, it may all seem a bit complicated. So let's get started.

The telltale sign of a new label is its heading, "Nutrition Facts", vs the old "Nutrition Information per Serving". Some of the changes include:

Serving size is now dictated by product line, and is a more realistic reflection of the amount people eat.

The list of nutrients covers those with which we should be the most concerned, including fat, cholesterol, dietary fiber, and sugars. No longer will thiamin, riboflavin and niacin be noted, as deficiencies of these vitamins are extremely rare. Sodium and iron are still listed.

Calories from fat are now shown, making it a bit easier to calculate the % of calories from fat. (calories from fat % total calories)

Nutrition Facts

Serving Size 1 cup (228g)
Servings Per Container 2

Amount Per Serving
Calories 250   Calories from Fat 110

	% Daily Value*
Total Fat 12g	**18%**
Saturated Fat 3g	**15%**
Cholesterol 30mg	**10%**
Sodium 470mg	**20%**
Total Carbohydrate 31g	**10%**
Dietary Fiber 0g	**0%**
Sugars 5g	
Protein 5g	

Vitamin A 4%	•	Vitamin C 2%
Calcium 20%	•	Iron 4%

*Percent Daily Values are based on a 2,000 calorie diet. Your daily values may be higher or lower depending on your calorie needs.

	Calories	2,000	2,500
Total Fat	Less than	65g	80g
Sat Fat	Less than	20g	25g
Cholesterol	Less than	300mg	300mg
Sodium	Less than	2,400mg	2,400mg
Total Carbohydrate		300g	375g
DietaryFiber		25g	30g

Calories per gram:
Fat 9   •   Carbohydrate 4   •   Protein 4

The larger labels will also include upper and lower limits of nutrients, assuming a 2000 or 2500 calorie per day diet. This part of the label will always be the same.

The % Daily Values tells you what % of a full day's nutrient requirement you are eating. Remember to keep your % of fat, especially saturated fat, and % DV cholesterol LOW, (you needn't reach 100%!) and your % of carbohydrates and dietary fiber HIGH. An important note: Hydrogenated oils, which react like saturated fats inside your body, are included in the Total Fats, but NOT included in the saturated fats. Watch for hydrogenated oils in your ingredients label. Also note that no % Daily Value has been set for sugars. We recommend 50 gms or less per day.

More good news is that many terms have been more specifically defined. For example, a food with a "Fat Free" claim can have no more than .5 gm fat per serving. "Low Fat" can have no more than 3 gm fat per serving. But remember, this applies only to individual foods. Entrees, like TV dinners, can have 3 gms for every 3.5 oz they weigh! So take Lean Cuisine's Meatloaf Dinner. With 9 total gms of fat, at 270 calories, 30% of its calories are from fat. Just make sure your total fat grams per day do not exceed 65.

LIGHT Foods contain 1/3 less calories or 1/2 less fat than their reference. Light sodium is half the normal content.

LEAN, when describing anything other than meat or poultry, is still rather nebulous. And even then you should buy "extra lean".

And last but certainly not least, certain claims may now be made linking a nutrient or food to the risk of a disease or health related condition. Is that not progress!?! Absolutely, positively, there IS a link between your diet and your health! Seven health messages are allowed:

- calcium and a lower risk of osteoporosis
- fat and a greater risk of cancer
- saturated fat and cholesterol and a greater risk of coronary heart disease
- fiber-containing grain products, fruits and vegetables and a reduced risk of cancer
- fruits, vegetables and grain products that contain fiber and a reduced risk of coronary heart disease
- sodium and a greater risk of high blood pressure
- fruits and vegetables and a reduced risk of cancer

If you feel a bit confused, remember, you are not alone. There is a lot of new information out there. The FDA offers a great brochure entitled "An Introduction to the New Food Label. They will also provide a seminar at your workplace explaining the new regulations, when available. In southern California call (213) 252-7597.

GOOD LUCK AND GOOD HEALTH!

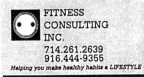

FITNESS CONSULTING INC.
714.261.2639
916.444-9355
Helping you make healthy habits a LIFESTYLE

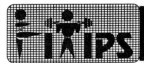

FITIPS August 1997

A study at the University of Illinois (Go Illini!) reveals people tend to eat more at each sitting from economy-sized snack packages. They surmise that we allow ourselves to consume more of a product when we believe that it is inexpensive and plentiful. So do yourself and your waistline a favor: Buy snack packs.

BIG Food

Many, many people over the past few decades have become more aware of their food choices. We are reading labels. We're counting fat grams. But studies reveal Americans are still getting fatter. In 1980, 25% Americans were considered obese. Today we're up to 30%. Could it possibly be our portions??

Let's first consider, what's a realistic "serving" size. Right or wrong, the USDA (US Dept. of Agriculture) provides us serving size recommendations for various foods. The FDA then requires that manufacturers provide these recommendations on all food labels. Let's compare those guidelines to reality...

The suggested serving size for a cola beverage is 8 oz. Canned beverages at 12 oz. are considered 1.5 servings. You might note at 7-11, however, you have "bigger" options. We've progressed from the "Gulp" at 16oz, to the Big Gulp at 32oz, to the Super Big Gulp with 44oz. And now we can indulge in 64oz of sugar-filled fluids with the Double Gulp. This 208 grams, or **52 teaspoons,** of nutrient-less sugar-water is _800_ calories!!! And _eight_ _times_ the recommended serving size!

Let's look at french fries. The recommended serving size is 3oz, which is 220 calories, equal to McDonalds small order. Get their Super Size and you consume 6oz and 440 calories.

Share a small box of theater popcorn with a friend and you will be close to consuming the recommended serving size of 24oz (3C). Share the large tub and you consume 65oz, or over double the endorsed amount. (Ever eat the whole box yourself?...)

Have you ever had a "bigger, better muffin"? Restaurants and bakeries often double the recommended serving size, giving you 4oz, or a quarter pound of flour, fat and sugar.

But maybe the USDA is unrealistic. Let's see what the American Heart Assn. has to say.

The American Heart Assn. recommends eating no more than 3-4 egg yolks/week. So one 3-egg omelette/week meets your quota.

They also suggest eating _no more_ than 6oz. of cooked lean meat, poultry or fish per day. Burger King's Double Whopper fills you with 1/2 lb, or 8oz, of meat. And not to be outdone, Carl's Jr's Double Western Bacon Cheeseburger has 1/2 lb meat **and** two strips of bacon! And did we mention hamburger is _not_ particularly "lean"??

Or how about kickin' up some dust at the local steakhouse. Despite the warnings about cholesterol and heart disease, the steak places claim bigger is better, with Mortons pride porterhouse at 48oz. (Eat 4oz. and take the rest home to enjoy over the next 11 days.)

So how do we escape this self-sabotaging trap?? Remember the **Dining OuTips**.

Here's to Lightening Up!!

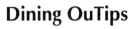

Dining OuTips

1. Share entrees with a friend.
2. Ask for a doggie bag, _especially_ at dinner.
3. Order entrees as your main course.
4. Eat more slowly. You'll feel full faster.
5. Focus on the dining experience and the company vs. over-emphasizing the food.

FITNESS CONSULTING INC.
Since 1985
Helping you make Healthy Habits a Lifestyle
(714) 261-2639

No Credit Cards!

The previous is a tough analogy
because in today's world, we rarely pay cash.

We are constantly using credit cards,
borrowing today with all good intentions of paying back tomorrow.

("I'd gladly pay you Tuesday for a hamburger today...")
[The original credit arrangement]

Unfortunately, the credit concept doesn't apply here.
We must keep within our daily budget - daily!

So how can I earn credits?

So you can't seem to stay within your budget??

That's a problem.

The good news is you <u>can</u> earn credits!

(whew!)

But you've got to <u>work</u> for them!

A half hour of aerobic exercise

ABOVE AND BEYOND YOUR PRESCRIBED DAILY AMOUNT

earns you 5 grams of fat.

So if your "daily debits"

exceed your daily budget,

you can work for more.

Once you put yourself on a

Fat Budget,

you quickly begin to look for ways to

SAVE!

So peruse our **SALE ADS**

for exciting Savings Ideas!

120

SALE

Get 10 extra grams

with a scenic bicycle ride

along the coast.

SAVE!!   SAVE!!   SAVE!!!

Save 5 fat grams

with a *BRISK* 30-minute

walk!!

EXTRA

SAVINGS!

Enjoy!
10 extra fat grams

with this invigorating

*Step Aerobics
Class!!*

SAVE 21 Grams!!

Breakfast of cereal, toast, & jam fruit & coffee

Only 4 grams!
(Regularly 25 with Sausage & Egg McMuffin)

SAVE! 10 grams!!

Bagel & Lite Cream Cheese

Only 5 Grams!
(Pastry normally 15 grams)

Pasta Salad

with onions, green peppers, carrots, kidney beans

Loaded with **Beta Carotene**

Only 6 grams of fat!

Beats a Taco Salad @ 66 grams!

Veggie Potato

w/ tuna salad & tomato
(NF mayo, please)

Only 2 Fat Grams!!

Avoid the cheese-laden spud @ 35 grams.

Drive Thru Savings

Grab a Grilled Chicken Sandwich
(vs. a messy burger)
and

SAVE 25-60 grams!

SAVE

Spaghetti Dinner

SAVE

w/ turkey meatballs
*includes salad w/ LF dressing, roll & honey

Only 10 Fat Grams

SAVE

Normally 58 w/ lasagna, fatty dressing & butter

SAVE

Exercise

Make several copies of the following Fat Register & maintain daily for a week.

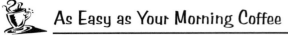

Fat Register

Date: _____

Date	Food	Fat Debit (-)	Exercise Credit (+)	Balance
				50 / 40

The Pantry Purge

There are no foods you can never eat.

There are some foods, however, that you <u>will</u>
eat if they are in your pantry, that have such *easy* substitutes,
and are so counter-productive
that you truly are better off throwing them away.
If you are committed to making more healthy choices
for both yourself and your family,
why keep this unhealthy stuff around?

It will just tempt you to eat it, then you will feel guilty afterwards.

So get out a big garbage bag.

Let's go...

real mayo
TV dinners over 25 grams of fat
crisco
ice cream
donuts   ding dongs   pork rinds   potato chips   muffins
high fat (Ritz) crackers

<u>Warning:</u> This exercise can be somewhat emotionally challenging.

<u>Ignore</u> your chatter that is saying, "But look at all the money I spent on that food!
I'll use them up and just not buy any more."

EATING THEM IS SELF DESTRUCTIVE, AND <u>NOT</u> WORTH THAT MONEY.

You may want to have a friend with you
for support, hand holding and perspective.

<u>**NOTE:**</u> This exercise has similar payoff to purging your closet.
Getting rid of all those old rags you no longer wear is invigorating and motivating.
You are on the road to new, more healthy choices.

Step #9

Moderate Sugar

Sugar is one of America's favorite foods. (Isn't it one of the four basic food groups?)

Cookies — pastries — cakes — ice cream. On average, we each consume 150 lbs per year. Now that's a <u>mound</u>!

For most people, there is nothing wrong with having a little bit of a sweet tooth. There is no conclusive evidence that there is any correlation between sugar intake in moderation and disease. Even diabetes is not caused by excessive sugar intake, though diabetics need to be cognizant of the amount of sugar they consume. In fact, if you earnestly tried to eliminate sugar from your diet, it would be nearly impossible, as most foods contain some sugar. Cereals — crackers — condiments — sauces.

So how did sugar get such a bad rap?

Well, it does have its pitfalls.

First, sugar often dances with fat, and fat IS bad for you. Our traditional cakes, cookies, and pies are loaded with both sugar and fats, often saturated. And we have discussed the hazards of saturated fats.

Trendy Nutrition: Juice Bars

Today's hot ticket is Juice Bars. No, not popcycles. Smoothies. Fruit and juice drinks, complete with yogurt and protein powder. The new and improved Breakfast of Champions. Get your daily dose of Vitamins in one fell swoop.

Well, guess what. That ain't all your're getting. Along with all that Vitamin A & C, you're taking in about 52 grams of sugar in a 32oz. smoothie.

<u>Double</u> your daily recommended amount.

So consider a smoothie for an occasional dessert. And get your morning Vitamins from a 1-a-Day.

Note: 1-a-day Vitamin $.10
         32oz smoothie $ 3.00

Secondly, sugar is essentially "empty calories", void of any nutritional value. No vitamins or minerals. (Though brown sugar has a little iron.) Just simple carbohydrates that convert to glucose, then into fat if not used as energy. (So if you are having a sugar craving, get your fix then go for a run...)

Sugar also makes you hungry. When you eat sugar, your blood sugar immediately rises. Then your pancreas secretes insulin into your blood stream to bring your sugars back down to normal levels, and it always over does it. So your blood sugar level drops below where it started. Then you feel hungry, feel a craving for sugar, grab another cookie or donut, and so the cycle continues.

And finally, sugar robs you of precious energy. Go back to the blood sugar "dips". When your insulin overreacts to the sugar you've eaten, it causes a blood sugar crash. Your energy then plummets. Your moods follow next, and soon you will begin to feel tired, lethargic and irritable. So drink a coke and you will feel energized for awhile, but soon comes the downfall. Same with morning pastries – or candy bars – or juice drinks.

Do things really go better with coke?

You may be saying to yourself right now, "This doesn't apply to me". You're not much of a cookies or candy kind of person.

So what is your favorite beverage with lunch?

Coke? Snapple? Hansons?

How about mid-day?

Another coke? Another Snapple?

So honestly, how often do you cruise the 7-11 for a Big Gulp?

A **Double Gulp**!?! That's 64 oz. of pure unadulterated sugar! About 50 teaspoons, to be not-so-exact! (Depends on your ice fetish.)

The average American consumes **150 pounds of sugar** each year. Are you ready for this? That comes out to 14,400 teaspoons per year, or nearly 40 teaspoons a day! (And you're worried about a couple tsp. on your breakfast cereal...?!) And much of this sugar comes in the form of corn syrup in beverages.

129

So What About Artificial Sweeteners?

Artificial Sweeteners have been on the market for decades, allowing us to temper our sweet teeth without the calories.

Wise choice?

Under the Universal Condition: All things in moderation. And in today's health conscious (or is it "Body Conscious"...?) world, that can be challenging.

Between the handful of "diet" colas we drink, coupled with the "diet" desserts and "diet" candy, our daily consumption of artificial chemicals − ugh − sweeteners can quickly become substantial. There is no information available on the long-term physical effects of over consumption because the products have not been on the market long enough.

I guess we will find out in another few decades...

<u>Alcohol</u>

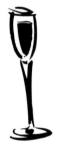
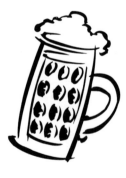

Alcohol is metabolized in your body much the same as sugar. The alcohol is converted to glucose, your blood sugar rises temporarily, then you crash.

This is one reason why we so often get the munchies after drinking.

For more information on alcohol, take a look at the following FiTips...

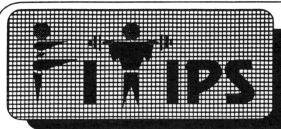

FiTips December 1993

* Manufactures Globulin, for sustaining your immune system.
* Manufactures Prothrombin, for blood clotting.
* The liver also detoxifies alcohol, and processes cholesterol and triglycerides.

"'Tis the Season to be Jolly..."

But all too often this translates into too much brew. As long as you have a designated driver, a few extra drinks on occasion are not a problem. But excess alcohol on a regular basis can create havoc with your insides. Following is a short anatomy lesson, describing the functions of a few of your organs, and the possible problems caused by alcohol:

Your **STOMACH's** normal function is food digestion, with the help of hydrochloric acids.

Alcohol Related Problems: Causes increases in production of acids, causing stomach lining to become irritated, inflamed, ulcerous, or potentially perforated. Vomiting is first symptom of irritation due to obstruction of passageway to intestine. Food has nowhere to go but **UP**.

SMALL INTESTINE's

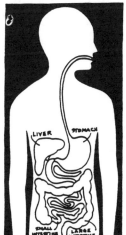

normal function is to continue the digestive process, and absorption of nutrients into the bloodstream.

Alcohol Related Problems: Slowed absorption of vitamins, plus increased excretion of vital minerals, including zinc, magnesium, and calcium.

PANCREAS normal function is manufacturing of digestive enzymes and insulin.

Alcohol Related Problems: Inflammation of pancreas causes digestive enzymes to be trapped inside, resulting in "digestion" of its internal lining. This condition is very painful, and sometimes fatal. Also, if the pancreas stops manufacturing insulin, diabetes occurs.

Normal **LIVER** functions include:
* Manufacture of bile, a digestive enzyme, from dead red blood cells.
* Manufactures Albumin, which maintains strong, healthy cells.

Alcohol Related Problems:
* Jaundice, due to excess dead red blood cells.
* Cell disintegration, from muscle, to brain, to heart cells.
* Weak immune system.
* Hemorrhaging from impaired clotting mechanism (this, coupled with tendency for bleeding ulcers in the stomach is a formula for disaster).
* Alcohol detoxifies more slowly, staying in your system longer, increasing its destruction. And Cholesterol and triglycerides increase in the bloodstream, increasing risk of heart disease.

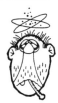

Alcohol also can be a contributor to psychological difficulties during the Holiday Season. It is a depressant, so just a few hours after consumption, you will begin to feel its negative effects. During a Season that can be inherently stressful anyway, alcohol can heighten your anxieties.

So when do you need to worry about these problems? How much is too much?

Experts define a drink as a 12 oz. beer, 4 oz. wine, or a shot of hard liquor. And *too much* is *more than two drinks a day.* Consider alcohol consumption as analogous to sun bathing. If you stay out for a few hours and your skin gets "pink", it quickly goes away with no real harm done. If you indulge for several hours, you likely will burn and peel. You actually lose skin cells, but your body makes new ones. If you have ever seen a survivor of a severe burn accident, however, you know his skin does not heal. It becomes permanently scarred. And so it is with your liver. "Burn" it with alcohol enough times, and it will become scarred and dysfunctional. Then you really have problems.

So this year, *enjoy* the Holidays. But remember to celebrate the miracle of the human body, rather than destroy it.

Happy, Healthy Holidays to You and Yours *

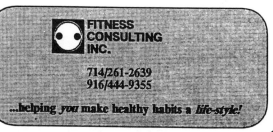

Where's the ~~Beef?~~ Sugar

If you are trying to locate sugar in your ingredients labels, remember it isn't always spelled S-U-G-A-R. It is very often called sucrose, fructose, glucose, dextrose, corn syrup, maple syrup, or even honey. But all these varieties of sugar are the same in terms of nutritional value. There is no credence to the myth that brown sugar or raw sugar, for example, are "better for you" than white sugar (sucrose). Your body metabolizes them all the same.

So **Buyer Beware!** As you read the ingredients label, looking for the "top 4"*, understand that though sugar may not be found at the top, the combination of all the varieties listed likely total a substantial amount.

Look at the following label.
What do you guess is the product?

Note: Ingredients are listed in descending order by volume, so the first ingredients listed are the most plentiful.

Mystery Product

Ingredients: sugar, wheat, corn syrup, honey, hydrogenated soybean oil, salt, caramel color, soy lecithin.

Answer: Kellogg's Smacks
(Formerly Sugar Smacks)
Understand why?

Sweet Treats

Got a Sweet Tooth?

Looking for something sweet, without loads of fat or sugar?

Try some of these low-fat sweet treats.

	sugar grams
Lowfat graham crackers with nonfat milk (just like kindy garten)	9
Snackwells chocolate chip cookies (13 o' those suckers! And "Got milk?" Get a serving of NF dairy to boot!)	10
Frozen grapes (1/2C) (Ever tried it?)	14
Half a peach over lowfat ice cream (1/2 C)	16
Cafe Mocha (nonfat) (Remember: Do decaf @ nite!)	5
Haagen-Dazs Chocolate Sorbet Bars	15
Hot apple sauce w/ cinnamon (1/2 C) (Look for the unsweetened.)	8
Baked Apple	21
Vanilla yogurt and berry parfait (1/2 C ea.) (Whew! Barely made it!*)	24

Remember: The recommended sugar limit is 25 grams/day.

Exercise

1. Try one of the Sweet Treats you have never tasted instead of the typical fat-filled dessert.

2. Limit your sweetened beverages to 12oz/day.

Step #10

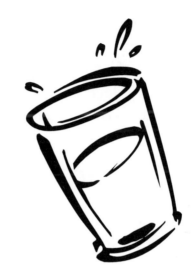

8 Glasses
of
Water/Day

Water, water everywhere...

...but cokes and coffee we drink.

Consuming 8 glasses of water a day is one of those recommendations of which we are all aware - and don't follow. From "I don't like the taste" to "it's too inconvenient to go potty so often", we have lots of excuses. So let's take a moment to refresh our memories on the "why for's" of water.

Remember, an adult's body weight is comprised of 55-65% water, with a 10% loss posing a significant health risk. Your body's need for water is second only to it's need for oxygen. (and you thought pizza was #2...) Water is the medium for all body fluids, including blood, the lymph, the digestive juices, urine and perspiration. It balances acids, moves nutrients into the cells, and is a solution for holding electrolytes (salts that allow the conveyance of electrical currents). And if that's not enough, drinking lots of water helps you lose weight! It increases your metabolism and your blood volume, making you a better fat burner.

So regular H20 stops should be a priority, especially in the summer months when temperature, and hopefully exercise, increase. This is especially true for those of you who work outside. Note that during physical activity only 25% of the energy generated by the body is turned into mechanical work, with the balance converted to heat. In order to keep your engine from overheating, the body is forced to sacrifice some of its valuable fluid reserves through sweating. If these are not replenished, you can become dehydrated, which can cause headaches, fatigue, and nausea.

And remember, don't wait until you are thirsty to drink. And don't stop drinking just because your thirst is quenched.

The call to consume the equivalent of 8 glasses of water per day includes all the food and beverages you take in throughout the day. Milk and other beverages are mostly water. Many foods have a high water content, especially fruits and veggies. Soups are also full of water. Remember that caffeinated and alcoholic beverages increase urination, but you do get some "water points" for them. When your urine is clear, you have had enough fluids.

Following are some tips for making the water challenge "do-able":

- Keep water with you during the day, especially if you are in and out of a vehicle.
- Keep a favorite mug or water glass at your desk.
- Add lemon or lime to enhance the flavor
- Start your day with a large glass of water, and drink a glass at every meal.
- Alternate your sodas and/or coffee with a glass of water.

BOTTOMS UP!

Exercise

Heeding the challenge to "Just Drink It",
condition yourself to drink some water
at each of the following times:

· every time you go potty

· each time you go to the copy machine

· whenever your pager goes off

· when the phone rings

Or program your computer to give you a

Water Break Reminder

on the hour.

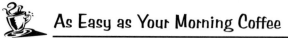
As Easy as Your Morning Coffee

Step #11

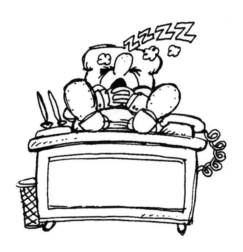

Rest

Conceptually, one of the benefits of technology is allowing us to accomplish more tasks in a shortened period of time. The net result, theoretically, is more discretionary and leisure time.

Right?

Wrong.

The ever-increasing pace of life today is dizzying. Faxes and phones and traffic and meetings and commitments and obligations and... and... and...

It never ends.

We are coming into work earlier, staying later, and working through lunch. It's no wonder the first words that come to mind when we consider starting a fitness program are,

" I just don't have time!!"

Then the weekends arrive, potentially an opportunity for a little "down time" – some R & R – maybe even a nap?

Nope.

Too busy.

Gotta do this. Gotta do that. Gotta go here. Gotta go there.

And quick as a flick the weekend is over and you are back at your desk - tired.

Nature's cycle constantly alternates between activity and rest - highs and lows - fast and slow. But we insist on staying in the fast lane, ignoring our body's need for rest.

Rest comes in two forms. First, sleep. How much do we need, and are there strategies for improving the restfulness of our sleep?

Sleep time is your body's opportunity to mend and restore itself. Cells and tissues are made and repaired. It is a time for healing and recovery from injuries or illness.

It's when your body's "internal elves" get all their maintenance work done...

Sleep is also a time for mental rejuvenation. Studies have revealed that volunteers going 2-4 days without sleep experience distortion, mood shifts and headaches. (Sounds like a normal day to me!...) When asked to execute physical tasks, however, the typical measures of physical exertion including blood pressure, heart rate, and oxygen uptake were not impacted by the sleep deprivation.

We have no clear determination of the number of hours sleep per night is necessary for good health. Some people feel best after 9-10 hours. Others only regularly need six. The important factor seems to be *quality* of sleep.

So following are some tips for heightening the quality of each night's sleep:

1. Exercise - Stanford University observed two groups of seniors, 50+ people who often experience sleep disruptions. Though both groups were sedentary at the start of the study, one group began exercising 30-40 minutes four times per week during the observation period. The active group reported sleeping an hour longer each night, and falling asleep more quickly.

2. Avoid Caffeine 2-4 hours before bedtime – Caffeine is a stimulant that will disturb sleep.

3. Avoid Cigarettes - The nicotine is a stimulant.

4. Avoid Excess Alcohol – As mentioned earlier, alcohol bounces your blood sugar and will disrupt sleep.

5. Maintain a Regular Sleep Schedule – If you must get up early, go to bed at your normal time anyway.

6. Control your Sleeping Environment – Keep your bedroom quiet, dark and a moderate temperature (60-65 degrees).

7. Relax Before Bedtime – Read. Listen to quiet music. Take a warm bath. (A hot bath is actually invigorating.) Avoid horror and high drama movies that excite your system.

8. Sex before bed is very relaxing!

Rest, however, is about more than just sleep.

It's about taking care of your body throughout the day.

It's about taking time to slow down – take a deep breath or two – regroup.

But not us we're too busy we've got so many important things to do and everything is a rush don't have time to stop eat on the run if at all planes to catch deadlines to meet meetings meetings meetings get to the bank kids to soccer who's got time to even go potty?

And so it goes...

Day after day.

Rush. Rush. Rush.

Ever get tired of rushing?

When was the last time you sat down and read a great novel? or took a long walk in the woods? or just sat at the beach and watched the waves?

No time?

Reconsider.

You need down time. Relaxation time is every bit as important as your aerobic exercise.

It's about balance.

It's about taking care of you...just for a short while.

Exercise

Following are some 1-minute, 5-minute, 30-minute, and 2-hour relaxation ideas. Add your own ideas to the list.

1-minute

close your eyes and breathe deeply

roll your shoulders

_____

_____

_____

_____

5-minute

take a brisk walk

stand up and stretch

read the funnies

draw cartoons

_____

_____

_____

_____

143

30-minute

- take a bubble bath

- take a nap

- watch a Lucy or Hogan's Heroes rerun

_____

_____

_____

_____

2 hours

- snuggle up with a good book

- watch an old movie

- go to the mall or an airport and "people watch"

_____

_____

_____

_____

We don't seem to have any shortage of great relaxation ideas,
it's just allowing ourselves to do them!

Exercise

Each day this week, take at least two breaks,
even if they are just for a minute.

Document them here.

Monday _____

_____

Tuesday _____

_____

Wednesday _____

_____

Thursday _____

_____

Friday _____

_____

Saturday _____

_____

Sunday _____

_____

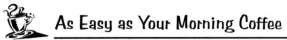

Step #12

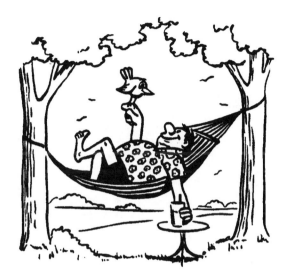

Let Go
of
Stress

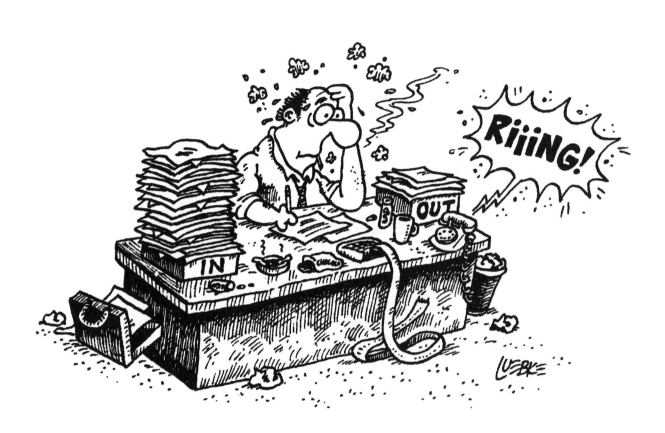

How's your body?

Stress is defined as "the importance or significance attached to a thing". Interesting. Because isn't stress caused by our attaching importance or significance to something?

Traffic is stressful because our <u>time</u> is valuable.

Money matters are stressful because all our <u>worldly attachments</u> are deemed valuable.

Relationships can be stressful because we feel it is important to be in control, to be right, to feel secure.

So what if we changed our perceptions of what we consider to be important?

The reality is traffic and money concerns and relationship struggles are all a part of life. They are not going to go away unless we move to a deserted island somewhere. Then we would feel stressed because we were bored.

So the key is to learn to manage these stressors; to actively choose to process them differently, avoid them, and/or treat stress's physical manifestations.

Don't go there

One of the easiest ways to avoid stressful situations is to avoid them. If traffic makes you crazy, choose to drive during non-peak traffic times. If financial stressors get you down, slow down your spending so it's no longer an issue. If time pressures cause you stress, assess your commitments and determine whether some need to disappear.

There is no question, we can simply avoid a number of common stressors.

Change Your Tapes

Our mental programming can also be a stressor.

Ever find yourself saying "I'm too fat!" or "I could never do that" or "I'm just not good enough"?

We sabotage ourselves with our negative chatter. We create stress because we talk ourselves into it. So don't go there, either. Instead, change the negative into positive self talk:

- I am consistently moving toward a more healthy lifestyle.
- I regularly try new things and whether or not I am successful, I always learn something.
- I am extremely talented in a variety of areas.

You may not believe these things about yourself initially, but KEEP SAYING THEM!

By reciting them to yourself day after day, soon you will believe it!

Release It

In the event you choose not to move to a deserted island and you are unsuccessful at ridding your life of stress, treating its symptoms becomes a critical health maintenance routine. And "routine" it should be. "A regular course of procedure; common practice; habitual; customary." This means more than a semi-annual weekend away. It means <u>daily</u>.

So what kinds of things can you do to get rid of stress? Following are a few suggestions.

Journaling

If you were asked to describe in writing what is bothering you, could you?

Would you?

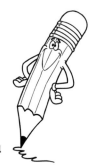

Journaling, or writing down your thoughts, has proven in many studies to be extremely therapeutic. It gives you the chance to be totally honest and unrestrained − to "tell it like it is" − and simply "getting it out" will make you feel better.

It also helps you to *process* the issue. If you allow yourself the time to write long enough, you can often move from the symptoms to the real problem. And understanding the problem and your feelings surrounding it is the first step toward resolution.

If you have never done journaling before, start out by answering the question,

How do I feel?

Then begin to honestly answer...

I feel pressured at work.

I don't feel appreciated.

I feel very nervous about my future...

Then expound as explicitly as possible.

I feel pressured at work. I'm not comfortable with my abilities to effectively do my job. My boss is always looking over my shoulder - micro-managing me. Maybe she isn't confident in my skills either.

But I really believe I <u>could</u> do the job, if only I understood her priorities. I feel so overwhelmed. Maybe I need to get organized. I could identify all the tasks she's asked me to complete, and ask her to prioritize them. She maybe doesn't even remember telling me to do all the things she's told me to do.

Maybe <u>she's</u> unorganized! Maybe if I identify all the tasks, get her input on priorities, I can relax and do them one at a time.

That's what I'll do!

Then I'll clean my house. I feel overburdened by all the responsibilities of owning a home...

...and so it goes.

Now obviously all difficult issues are not going to be resolved via journaling. But your <u>feelings</u> can be identified and acknowledged, which will make you feel better.

Let's try it.

How am I feeling?

Exercise

One of the best stress management techniques is exercise. Getting physical – elevating your heart rate – is a great way to "get it out of your system". You will always **feel** better after exercising, whether or not the issue gets resolved. Then you will be in a better position to deal with the problem.

And there is a physiological reason for you feeling better. After several minutes of aerobic exercise, your body produces endorphines, or "happy chemicals" that make you feel good and positive. These same chemicals are manufactured by your body during laughter. So it is an exercise-induced "happy drug".

Eat

Next time you are feeling stressed and irritable, look at your gas gauge. When was the last time you stopped to have a bite to eat? Several hours? Remember, food is your friend. It's your fuel. Eating regularly keeps your blood sugar consistent which will help to combat the day's challenges.

Breathe and Stretch

When you are in the middle of a stressful day and cannot leave to go for a run, don't underestimate the power of breathing and stretching.

Sit with your eyes closed and take long (15-30 second*) deep breaths, each time completely filling your belly. Exhale very slowly. Within 3 minutes you will lower your pulse rate and blood pressure.

Your body has an amazing capability to heal and nurture itself. Allowing yourself to STOP the chaos, close your eyes, and breathe for even 3 minutes 2-3 times/day will significantly reduce stress and its physical effects.

When you are stressed, your body's natural response is to tense up. So a difficult day often is followed by a sore neck, shoulders and back.

Don't let it get ya!

Combat it throughout the day with some simple neck, shoulder and back stretches. (See Step #4)

* only in America is 15 seconds considered a "long time"...

Brain Stray

Finding ourselves in situations we don't want to be in creates stress. Be it traffic, too many commitments, or financial woes, stress is a reaction to an unpleasant situation.

So "go on vacation". Put yourself into an alternative "story". Disappear. And anything is possible in your mind.

Read a Fairy Tale and become The Queen. (Or maybe you are more interested in being the Wicked Witch...)

Then write your own ending to the story:

· Maybe you put the source of your frustrations "in the dungeon".

· Maybe dyno-birds carry him away...

· or lions eat him...

· or she has to polish Cinderella's shoes...

Whatever the end of your story, it is sure to make you feel better.

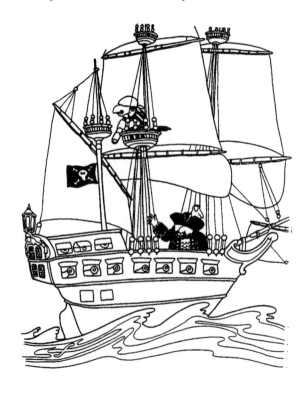

Play is O.K.

One of the cool things about kids is you can **play** with them. If you are on the floor with a 3-year old playing

Vvvrrrroooooom!

with race cars, everyone thinks it is noble of you to take the time to entertain the child.

HA! You think it's great! You haven't been able to play with cars since you were a kid!

The classic example of this truth is the child watching Daddy play with his train set at Christmas, and the child barely gets a shot at it! Daddy's having too much fun!

But the bummer is, unless there is a child present, it is not socially acceptable for adults to play.

Very sad.

Playing is good for the soul.

Being childlike.

Free from constraints.

Laughing.

When was the last time you let yourself go and acted childlike?

Can you even remember?!

As a result, you may need to work into this one slowly. You may not feel immediately compelled to *skip* down Main St.

But take small steps.

Wear a silly hat.

Place a funny character on your desk.

Play the kazoo for someone's birthday.

Then step a little further out on a limb:

- fly a kite

- try the hoola hoop

- blow soap bubbles

- or bubble gum bubbles. – **Grape** – Two or three pieces at once!

Then when you really get into it you'll be inviting friends to "come out and play". And you'll be having so much fun you won't even notice their utterly strange looks.

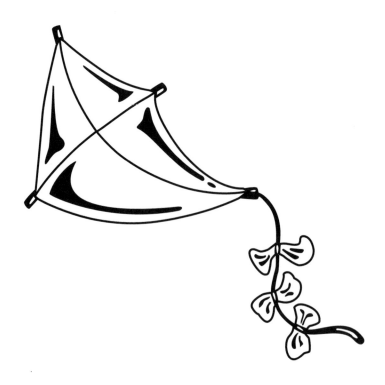

Why Don't We Play?

Probably because we are too busy being adults, and that's "serious business". Don't the rules say that after a certain age, we are to "act like adults", suggesting adults don't play any more?

Honestly, Dads, how would you feel if your 17 year old son were still playing with toy race cars? Or your teenage daughter was still dressing dolls? It's just not acceptable behavior.

We are also concerned about "looking silly". We do have an image to keep, you know.

If you are a teenager, you must look cool. As men mature, they must look macho, professional, suave, and/or sophisticated. Girls and women want to look attractive, sophisticated, and/or ladylike. And it truly is tough to look sophisticated with grape bubble gum all over your face.

There is a time and a place and a purpose for all these behaviors and boxes. (How much work would we get done if Corporate America began donning silly noses and big ears - blowing bubbles down the corridor...) But be sure to let yourself <u>out</u> once in awhile! It's good for the soul!

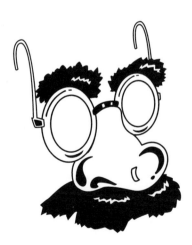

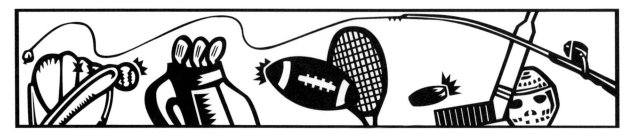

Sports as Play

Sports are one way adults play.

And therapeutic it is!

How fun is a rousing game of softball or shooting a little "hoop".

And tell me you don't regress to your childhood
when you are going kamikaze down a hill on your mountain bike?

But Sportsters Beware!

Take it <u>not</u> too seriously!

All too often we become so competitive, even in our play,
that play becomes serious and ceases to be play.

ENJOY the process!

Relish the Play!

Have fun!

You'll be glad you did.

Exercise

Do one of the following, or choose your own mode of play, then do some journaling about how it made you feel.

- Peruse a toy store.

- Read a Fairy Tale.

- Play jacks or hop scotch.

- Climb a tree.

- Eat a popcycle.

- Go on a Ferris Wheel.

- Color, either in a coloring book, or create your own.

- Swing.

_____

_____

_____

_____

_____

_____

_____

The
Last
Chapter

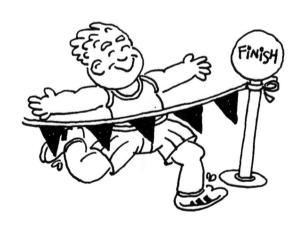

Back to the Numbers

Early in this process I encouraged you to "look at the numbers."

We discussed the difference between body fat percentage and weight.

You began taking your pulse regularly, understanding it's correlation to your heart getting stronger.

You even became aware of the number of push-ups you could do.

So, how are you doing?

One of the greatest rewards for establishing healthier habits is watching your body respond.

It's motivating to see your cholesterol go down.

It's exciting to see muscles appear.

It's a rush to watch your resting heart rate get lower and lower.

So pay attention!

Continue to keep track of these numbers.

Test and retest and retest. Make a quarterly appointment with your Fitness Consultant **and <u>keep it</u>!** (makes a difference...)

Keep your Fitness Record up to date.

It keeps you on track.

It keeps you motivated.

It keeps you accountable.

Just like any other goal with a plan,

you must regularly monitor your progress along the way.

How are you feeling?

The last several weeks you have made some key changes in your lifestyle and habits.

You have eaten more veggies. (Do you feel like you are turning into a veggie?!?)

You are moving more.

You feel better about yourself.

Right?

You must decide

In order for any program to be successful long-term, it must be "working". In order to sustain your commitment, (and a *commitment* it is...) you must be <u>convinced</u> it is worth the return.

So... is it?...

One Last Exercise

(I promise...)

Do some journaling about how you are feeling about the changes you have made in your life.

Have they been positive? Negative?

Where do you want to go from here?

_____

_____

_____

_____

_____

_____

_____

_____

The End?

You did it! You made it through all 12 Steps!

Now what?!?

Keep on keepin' on.

Self care is an ongoing, lifelong process. It's not like painting a picture, where you're finished when you finish. You must commit to taking care of yourself for a lifetime. Because if you don't, who will?

You no longer have Mr. P.E. Teacher monitoring your exercise.

Mom doesn't keep track of your food any longer.

If you are stressed out, who'll care?

YOU must take care of you.   Daily.   One step at a time.

It's kinda like brushing your teeth. It's a daily thing. It's something you commit to on a regular basis. You don't say, "I just don't have time to brush my teeth." You do it. *Daily.*

Give each of these steps the same commitment.

Commit to taking care of you. **Every** day.

All of us at Fitness Consulting sincerely wish you **_well_**.

Epilogue

Per a client request, I completed this book in time for an October 1997 engagement in Winnipeg. Two months later I learned I had thyroid cancer.

That was quite a shock for little Miss "Eats Perfectly, Exercises Regularly" Fitness Cheerleader. But like most experiences in life, lessons flourished.

The first and most obvious is there are no guarantees in life. You may think you are right on track – doing all the right things – and the gods decide you need a lesson. Guess what...you will be given the opportunity to learn a lesson.

Second, stress debilitates. Make all the excuses you want, "But it's only temporary...", "We need the money right now...", "I enjoy the stress...", "As soon as I......", stress debilitates. Let it go long enough and your body will let you know it's not happy about it.

Third, you <u>can</u> overcome. My process was surgery January 20, 1998, thyroid medication for four weeks, then <u>no</u> meds for two weeks. They wanted to starve my body of those hormones in preparation for taking a radioactive pill to obliterate any remaining cancer cells. I was told that during that two week period without meds I would be tired, lethargic, cold, and would certainly gain weight. Well, I decided I wasn't interested in any of that, and I'd do my very best to combat it. I continued to exercise 4-5 times per week, including both cardiovascular exercise and weight training. I logged all of my food – eating regularly and clean. And all the while I kept looking over my shoulder wondering when all the fatigue was going to set in.

Bottom line: Days 12-14 I was a little more tired. Day 15 I fell in the black hole. (Couldn't get warm on a 70° Southern California day; slept all afternoon) And then I climbed back out – and never looked back. My weight at my last doctor's visit was 3lbs. less than my first visit. (Though we <u>know</u> weight is irrelevant!) So when you're up against a physical challenge:

1. <u>Decide</u> to overcome – attitude is everything

2. Take care of your body and it will take care of you.

Lastly, and absolutely not least, I needed to learn the power of community. For most of my adult life I described myself as "independent to a fault", not sincerely believing the "fault" part. So when I was told I had cancer and my family tried to surround me, my natural response was "It's no big deal." ... "Doctor says I'll just be tired." ... "I can take care of myself." ... "I'll be ok." Luckily, they didn't listen to me. Sister Jane flew out to be with me for the week. I received calls and e-mails (Isn't e-mail terrific!?) from across the country. My house looked like a funeral parlor. What became crystal clear is independence can be a disease. We need community – love – touch – support – family. So if you're shunning your support team, remember Step #13 is "Cherish your Community".

About the Author

Judi Ulrey is the founder and owner of Fitness Consulting, Inc., a southern California based provider of Corporate Wellness Programs. Since 1985 their motto has been "Helping you make healthy habits a *lifestyle*", and their mission is to get people moving, eating well, and taking care of themselves. Their services include:

- Health/Fitness Education
- Fitness Testing
- On-site Activity Classes
- Corporate Fitness Center Management

Judi also travels nationally and internationally speaking to a variety of audiences on the benefits of self care. Due to her strong belief in and passion for her topic, she consistently receives very high ratings. For more information on Judi's seminars, call us at (949) 644-1202, or check out our web site at www.fitnessconsulting.com.

Judi and all her staff sincerely hope this book will be helpful in your process.

Special Note

In several places throughout this book you will find reductions of our newsletter, "FiTips".

FiTips has been an integral part of Fitness Consulting's educational program for our corporate clients. Each month we bring a new fitness topic to the employees' attention. From Best Fast Foods to Blood Pressure Basics, we try to keep fitness front of mind through this creative, informal newsletter. I hope you enjoy reading them!

And if you would like more information on a subscription for your company, church, school, etc. just give us a call at (949) 644-1202, or find us at www.fitnessconsulting.com.

Enjoy!!

Appendix
(Orphan pages...)

Grocery List

General

Chicken
Fish
Lean Beef
Tuna
Tofu
Cottage Cheese
Lowfat Cheese
NF/LF Yogurt
Eggs
Milk - nonfat for drinking
       - 2% for coffee
NF/LF Sour Cream
Lotsa fruit
Lotsa veggies
Whole Wheat Bread\Bagels
Cereals (low sugar)
·   Cheerios
·   Grape Nuts
·   All Bran
·   Oatmeal
·   Raisin Bran
·   Cream of Wheat
Juice

Dried Goods

Pasta
Rice
Beans
Crackers -   Ak Mak
      -   Ry Krisp
      -   Melba toast
      -   Nabisco Harvest Crisps

Condiments

NF/LF mayo
Mustard
BBQ Sauce
NF/LF Salad Dressings
Balsamic Vinegar
Seasoned Rice Vinegar

Canned Goods

Beans - pinto
       - garbonzo
       - kidneys

Corn
Soups - 98% fat free cream of chicken/mushroom
       - lentil
       - bean/pea
Tomatoes/Tomato sauce
Fat Free chicken broth

Frozen Foods

Veggies - corn, peas, mixed
Sweet Treats - NF yogurt, LF ice cream, popcycles
    (gotta have somethin' for your sweet tooth...)
Whole Wheat Waffles

Other:

Hummus
Apple Sauce
Pasta Sauce

Kitchen Basics

Freezer Bags
Veggie Bags
Rice Cooker
Crock Pot
Food Processor (optional, but it helps
<u>tremendously</u> w/ weekly veggie chop-chop)

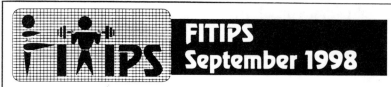

**FITIPS
September 1998**

Food Prep Made *Easy*

One of the biggest hurdles to eating well is <u>TIME</u>. Going out for lunch is easier than bringing it from home. Grabbing a bag of chips for dinner or cruising the drive-thru on your way home is faster than taking the time to fix something. But if you do a little prep on Sunday, your coming week will be easier and more healthy. Take a look:

1. **Fix one entree** and use it throughout the week. Chili over pasta one night and over a potato another gives you 2/5 meals. Throw it in your lunchbox one day and you've maxed your "chili efficiency". Or pasta salad with kidneys and lotsa veggies is easy to throw in your lunchbox as a side dish all week. (recipe in box)

2. **Chop your veggies.** If you have a food processor, this is a quick & easy task. Now you are ready to easily throw together a salad, or munch before dinner with some nonfat/lowfat ranch dressing. (Better choice than potato chips...) You can even pre-baggie them for your lunchbox.

3. **Boil a dozen.** Egg whites are a terrific protein source, so have them ready to throw in your salads.

4. **Bake your bird** (or parts of choice). Now it's ready to put in your tacos, salads, or quickly throw together chicken salad for sandwiches. (Remember to use nonfat or lowfat mayo...)

5. **Cook your grains.** The FDA recommends we eat 6-11 servings of whole grains a day, but the 45 minute cooking process is overwhelming on most evenings, and certainly for lunch. So do due diligence on Sunday and enjoy your carbos all week.
<u>Note</u>: A rice cooker is a <u>wonderful</u> investment!

Easy Pasta Salad

Boil your multi-colored spirels and chop-chop your multi-colored veggies (red, green & yellow peppers, red onion, colored zucchinis). In small bowl, mix 1/2C. nonfat or lowfat mayo, 2T. vinegar, and one can 98% fat free Cream of Celery Soup. Combine all of the above, finally adding kidneys and frozen peas. Yummy!

---

6. **Chunk your cheese.** If you have been successful in transitioning to nonfat cheese, "untraditional" cheese and crackers are A-OK. So cut your cubes for your lunch munch in the days ahead.

Making healthy food choices throughout the week <u>without</u> a lot of hassle is also dependent upon strategic grocery shopping for "grab-and-go" snacks. Make sure the following make it into your cart:

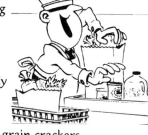

* baby carrots
* sweet peas
* lotsa fruit, especially the no-prep variety (bananas, cherries, apples, pears, plums)
* lowfat, whole grain crackers (reduced fat triscuit, ak mak, nonfat ry krisp, Snack Well's, wasa or melba)
* nonfat/lowfat yogurt
* snack pack cottage cheese (Great for cracker dipping!)
* whole wheat bagels (Don't forget the lite cream cheese!)
* dried fruit - raisins, apricots, prunes...
* pretzels
* pop-top tuna packed in water
* pop-top porky beans
* pop-top *unsweetened* apple sauce and pineapple
* dehydrated soup cups*
* dehydrated potato cups
* dehydrated cereal cups

So the key to success is:

<u>Prepare</u> for Battle!

* Don't overdo the "just add water" concept or you'll overdo your sodium.

 FITNESS CONSULTING INC.
Since 1985

Helping you make Health Habits a Lifestyle
(949) 261-2639

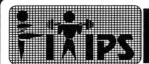

FITIPS August 1996

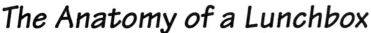

The Anatomy of a Lunchbox

Many of us spend the majority of our weekday waking hours at our workplace. Are you strategically planning your daytime foods, or leaving your fuel choices to the "luck of the lunch truck"? Remember, if you are eating foods you have prepared at home, you have much more control, and it is likely to be healthier.

The most logical lunchbox choice is leftovers from last night's dinner. Purposely prepare larger quantities so you can take them the next day for lunch. In fact, before dinner is served, pull out and pack lunch away, as "lunch" may not be left if you wait. Then it's ready to grab tomorrow.

Sunday afternoons/evenings are another lunch preparation opportunity. Cut up your veggies. (You are then more likely to eat

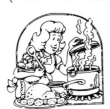

them during the week.) Make a dozen **burritos** and put them in the freezer. Make a pan of **lazagna**, cut it into squares, and freeze in individual portions. **Chicken and noodles** is another excellent Sunday afternoon prep that makes the following week's lunches a breeze. See the EASY recipe below. And if you make a pot of **chili,** one day you put it over a potato, the next over pasta, the third over rice. If you've done a little work ahead of time, you can "grab-and-go" during the week.

Remember the importance of eating "top heavy" for weight control purposes, meaning the majority of your calories (70%) should be consumed in the early and mid part of your day. A lunchbox greatly helps you do this. Bring 1000 calories worth of "good stuff" with you to work, and simply nibble all day. The result is your blood

sugar (as well as your moods...) maintain a consistent level, and you have consumed the calories you need during the active part of your day. Voalla!! Good-bye body fat!

Following are some low-fat lunchbox ideas:

- fruit
- veggies
- whole grain crackers w/ NF cream cheese*
- NF bean dip (use w/ crackers, veggies, pita bread...)
- Non- or low-fat yogurt
- Pasta Salad w/ chicken, tuna, or beans (add veggies and NF Ranch/Italian dressing, OR mix reduced fat cream of celery soup, 1/2C NF mayo & 2T of vinegar)
- Sandwich - turkey
           - lean ham
           - tuna
  Use NF mayo and lots of tomato and sprouts!

Chicken & Noodles, 1-2-3

1. Bake chicken. Let cool, and cut into pieces.

2. Cook "No Yolks" egg noodles.

3. Combine 1 & 2, and cover with a can of low fat cream of chicken soup.

Pepper to taste.

Scrumptious!

- Potato - Nuke @ the office & cover w/ salsa, cottage cheese, and/or NF sour cream.
- pretzels
- apple sauce (its a "fruit"!)
- soup or chili
- cup-o-soups (black bean over a potato, Mmmmm...)
- beans, rice and veggies, w/ lotsa salsa
- sweet treats: NF fig newtons, graham crackers, Snack Wells cookies
  Note: It is better to eat a little lunchtime sugar than a LOT of after dinner sugar...

* mix sun dried tomatoes, fresh basil and scallions, or fresh strawberries to your cream cheese for added zip.

FITNESS CONSULTING INC.
Since 1985
Helping you make Healthy Habits a Lifestyle
(714) 261-2639

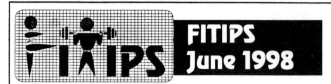

FITIPS June 1998

DRIVE-THRU "Do's & Don'ts"

You're short on time so you're cruisin' the drive-thru. Is there anything there you can eat with a clear health conscience?

Absolutely!! In meeting the demands of people interested in eating more consciously, Fast Food has come a long way! Look below at the good, the bad, and the UGLY!

Boston Market

Skinless Rotisserie	cal.	tot. fat.	%cal/fat	sod.(mg)
Turkey Breast	170	1	5%	850
Chicken Pot Pie	750	34	41%	2380
Ham w/ apples	350	13	33%	1750
Ceasar side salad	210	17	73%	560
Parmesan Creamed Spinach	280	21 (ouch!)	90%	820

Sides under 5gm fat:
Steamed veggies
Dill new potatoes
Cranberry walnut relish
Hot cinnamon apples
Herbed sweet corn
Rice pilaf
Corn bread
BBQ baked beans

Dairy Queen

	cal.			
Chicken Strip Basket*	1000	50	45%	2260
Chicken Breast Fillet Sandwich	430	20	42%	760
Grilled Chicken Sandwich	310	10	29%	1040
DQ Ultimate Burger	670	43	58%	1210
Med Choc Chip Cookie Dough Blizzard	950	36	34%	660
DQ soft serve choc. cone	150	5	30%	70

* Includes four breaded chicken strips, medium french fries, Texas toast & gravy. Consume only after your will is in order.

Taco Bell

	cal.	tot. fat	%cal/fat	sod.(mg)
Grande Burrito	420	22	47%	1050
Veggie Fajita	420	19	41%	920
Nachos Bell Grande	740	39	47%	1200
Lt. Chicken Soft Taco	180	5	25%	590
Taco Salad	840	52 (wow!)	56%	1670
Chicken Club	540	31	52%	1290

McDonalds

Big Mac	560	31	50%	1070
Fish Fillet	560	28	45%	1060
Gr. Chicken	440	20	41%	1040
Super FF	540	26	43%	350
Saus Bis/egg	510	35	62%	1210

Hardees

Bacon Chbgr	690	46	60%	1150
Gr. Chicken	350	11	28%	950
Ham & Ch	310	12	46%	1410
Rst. Beef	320	16	45%	820

> Don't miss this great fast food web site!
>
> www.olen.com/food/

Subway has done a fabulous job in offering quick, healthy options. They have seven sandwiches under six grams of fat, using lowfat cheese, mayo and meats. Yum!

For all of our Southern California readers, don't miss **Koo Koo Roo**. Loads of low fat side dishes, including cracked wheat rice, yams, lentil salad and roasted garlic potatoes. But steer clear of the turkey pot pie - 905 calories and 45 gm. fat!

Remember the daily fat intake guidelines:

Ladies, 35-45gm/day
Gentlemen, 45-55gm/day

Grab a Big Mac and you're pert near done!

Happy Healthy Dining!

 FITNESS CONSULTING INC.
Since 1985
Helping you make Healthy Habits a Lifestyle
(949) 261-2639